I0841320

Title: Harnessing AI for Anxiety Relief: A Comprehensive Guide for Sufferers (ISBN: 9798861702614)

Disclaimer: The information provided in this book is intended for informational and guidance purposes only. It is not a substitute for professional advice, diagnosis, or treatment. The author and publishers of this book shall not be held liable for any damages or consequences arising from the use or misuse of the information contained herein.

The content of this book is focused on utilizing AI to assist individuals with anxiety. While efforts have been made to ensure the accuracy and reliability of the information presented, the author and publishers do not guarantee the completeness, adequacy, or currency of the content.

It is important to note that the use of AI or any other techniques discussed in this book should always be done in consultation with licensed health professionals. Each individual's situation is unique, and decisions regarding treatment or management of anxiety should be made in partnership with qualified professionals who can consider the specific circumstances and needs of the individual.

Furthermore, the author and publishers do not endorse any specific AI tools, applications, or technologies mentioned in this book. The inclusion of such information is purely for illustrative purposes and does not constitute an endorsement or recommendation.

Readers are advised to exercise their own discretion and judgment when applying the information provided in this book. It is recommended to seek professional advice and conduct further research to ensure that any decisions made align with the individual's specific requirements and comply with applicable laws and regulations.

By reading this book, you acknowledge that you have read and understood this disclaimer, and you agree to release the author and publishers from any liability associated with the use or implementation of the information provided herein.

ISBN: 9798861702614

Note: The contents of this book were mainly produced by AI means, and thus, you will find that some of the content is not written in the format you would normally expect to find. However, you will find this book possesses a great deal of information that addresses almost every possible aspect of anxiety and what AI resources there are available to help you, your family, friends, patients, and students deal with anxiety. Names and links to resources are often listed in this book, but even if they are not, we encourage you to conduct your own searches using AI or other means to find resources that align with the suggestions listed in the chapters. The intention of creating this book was not to make a million dollars from those suffering from anxiety, as the curator of this material is a sufferer as well. I truly know how bad and debilitating anxiety can be, and I feel this book is in many ways, a quick reference to an alternative yet parallel way that people with anxiety can learn to cope with and, in ways, conquer its debilitating and paralyzing effects.

This book was created using AI software, but it still took a very long time to put the information together to ensure it was of value to readers. Given that the content was created using AI generative means, the price is much less than you would normally expect for a book like this. However, we firmly believe that if you approach using this book as a guide to further self-exploration, you will undoubtedly be on the road to finding information and approaches to greatly improve your quality of life.

Introduction:

Welcome to "Harnessing AI for Anxiety Relief: A Comprehensive Guide for Sufferers." This book is designed to provide valuable insights and practical guidance on how artificial intelligence (AI) can be utilized to support individuals struggling with anxiety. In an increasingly digital world, AI presents unique opportunities to enhance mental health care and provide personalized assistance to those in need.

Opening Address:

Dear Reader,

I am delighted to present this comprehensive guide, which aims to empower anxiety sufferers with knowledge and resources to navigate their journey towards relief. Anxiety can be a challenging and overwhelming condition, impacting various aspects of one's life. However, with the advancements in AI technology, we now have a new frontier of possibilities to explore.

In this book, we will delve into the potential applications of AI in anxiety management. We will explore how AI-powered tools, techniques, and interventions can complement traditional therapies, providing individuals with additional support and resources. It is important to note that this book does not replace professional advice or treatment; rather, it serves as a supplementary resource to inform and empower those seeking relief.

Throughout the chapters, we will discuss various AI-driven approaches, such as chatbots, virtual assistants, and machine learning algorithms, that can aid in anxiety management. We will explore their benefits, limitations, and ethical considerations to ensure a well-rounded understanding of their potential impact.

It is crucial to emphasize that the information provided in this book is intended for informational and guidance purposes only. Each person's experience with anxiety is unique, and what works for one individual may not work for another. Therefore, it is essential to consult with licensed health professionals to tailor strategies and interventions to your specific needs.

I encourage you to approach this book with an open mind, ready to explore the possibilities that AI offers in the realm of anxiety relief. Let us embark on this journey together, as we explore the intersection of technology and mental health, seeking innovative solutions to alleviate anxiety and improve overall well-being.

Wishing you a transformative and enlightening reading experience.

Sincerely,

Fellow Sufferer and Thriver

Table of Contents:

1. Understanding Anxiety: Causes, Symptoms, and Impact – page 8

2. Exploring the Role of AI in Anxiety Management – page 9

3. Benefits and Limitations of AI in Anxiety Relief – page 10

4. Getting Started: Setting Up Your AI Tools and Resources – page 11

5. Finding the Right AI-Based Anxiety Support Systems – page 14

6. Personalizing Your AI Experience: Tailoring AI Tools to Your Needs – page 15

7. AI-Powered Relaxation Techniques: Unwinding with Virtual Assistance – page 15

8. Cognitive Behavioral Therapy (CBT) with AI: Rewiring Your Thoughts – page 17

9. Identifying Anxiety Triggers: AI Insights for Self-Awareness – page 18

10. AI Chatbots: 24/7 Support for Anxiety Relief – page 20

11. AI-Enhanced Meditation and Mindfulness Practices – page 21

12. Tracking and Analyzing Anxiety Patterns with AI – page 23

13. AI-Driven Journaling: Expressive Therapy for Anxiety – page 26

14. AI-Powered Sleep Solutions: Restoring Peaceful Nights – page 27

15. Virtual Reality (VR) and Augmented Reality (AR) for Anxiety Management – page 30

16. AI-Enabled Biofeedback: Monitoring and Regulating Anxiety Symptoms – page 32

17. Ethical Considerations in AI-Based Anxiety Support – page 35

18. Integrating Human Connection with AI Support Systems – page 37

19. Combining Traditional and AI Approaches for Holistic Anxiety Relief – page 39

20. AI and Professional Therapy: Collaborative Care for Anxiety – page 42

21. Overcoming Stigma: Addressing Concerns about AI-Based Support – page 44

22. Evaluating the Effectiveness of AI Tools for Anxiety Relief – page 46

23. Navigating Privacy and Security in AI-Driven Solutions – page 48

24. AI and Self-Care: Integrating Healthy Habits into Your Routine – page 50

25. AI-Powered Anxiety Apps: A Comprehensive Review – page 52

26. AI in Wearable Technology: Monitoring and Managing Anxiety on the Go – page 55

27. AI and Social Support: Building Online Communities for Anxiety Relief – page 57

28. AI-Enhanced Breathing Exercises: Harnessing the Power of Deep Breathing – page 60

29. AI and Medication Management: Ensuring Safe and Effective Treatment – page 63

30. AI in Cognitive Training: Boosting Mental Resilience – page 66

31. AI for Anxiety Prevention: Identifying Early Warning Signs – page 68

32. AI in Workplace Wellness: Reducing Anxiety in Professional Settings – page 71

33. AI and Gamification: Making Anxiety Relief Engaging and Fun – page 74

34. AI and Nutrition: Enhancing Mental Well-being through Smart Food Choices – page 77

35. AI and Exercise: Motivating Physical Activity for Anxiety Relief – page 79

36. AI and Positive Psychology: Cultivating Optimism and Gratitude – page 81

37. AI and Mind-Body Practices: Balancing Energy and Emotions – page 84

38. AI and Virtual Support Animals: Finding Comfort in Digital Companions – page 86

39. AI and Music Therapy: Soothing Sounds for Anxiety Relief – page 89

40. AI and Art Therapy: Expressive Creativity for Emotional Healing – page 91

41. AI and Nature Therapy: Virtual Escapes to Calm the Mind – page 94

42. AI and Stress Management: Techniques for Tackling Everyday Stressors – page 96

43. AI and Trauma Recovery: Supporting Healing and Resilience – page 99

44. AI and Phobia Treatment: Overcoming Fears with Virtual Exposure – page 102

45. AI and Panic Attack Management: Coping Strategies at Your Fingertips – page 105

46. AI and Social Anxiety: Building Confidence in Social Settings – page 108

47. AI and Generalized Anxiety Disorder: Tools for Chronic Anxiety
– page 111

48. AI and Post-Traumatic Stress Disorder (PTSD): Aiding
Recovery – page 113

49. AI and Obsessive-Compulsive Disorder (OCD): Breaking Free
from Intrusive Thoughts – page 115

50. The Future of AI in Anxiety Relief: Innovations and Possibilities
– page 117

Note: Each chapter will provide a comprehensive overview of the
topic, practical tips, case studies, and recommendations for AI tools

Chapter 1: Understanding Anxiety: Causes, Symptoms, and Impact

Title: Introduction to Anxiety

Subtitle: A Comprehensive Guide

Anxiety is a common mental health condition that affects millions of
people worldwide. In this chapter, we will delve into the causes,
symptoms, and impact of anxiety. By understanding anxiety at a
deeper level, you will be better equipped to navigate its challenges
and explore ways to manage it effectively.

Causes of Anxiety:

Anxiety can arise from a variety of factors, including genetic
predisposition, environmental stressors, traumatic experiences, and
imbalances in brain chemistry. It is essential to recognize that
anxiety is not a personal failure or weakness but a complex interplay
of various factors.

Symptoms of Anxiety:

Anxiety manifests differently in individuals, but common symptoms include persistent worry, restlessness, irritability, difficulty concentrating, muscle tension, and sleep disturbances. It is crucial to identify these symptoms early on to seek appropriate support and intervention.

Impact of Anxiety:

Living with anxiety can significantly impact various aspects of life, including relationships, work or academic performance, and overall well-being. The constant presence of anxiety can be overwhelming and hinder one's ability to enjoy life to the fullest. However, there is hope. With the right tools and strategies, anxiety can be managed effectively, allowing individuals to regain control and lead fulfilling lives.

Chapter 2: Exploring the Role of AI in Anxiety Management

Title: Types of Anxiety Disorders

Subtitle: Understanding the Spectrum

Anxiety disorders encompass a range of conditions, each with its unique characteristics and challenges. By familiarizing yourself with different types of anxiety disorders, you can gain a better understanding of your own experiences or those of your loved ones.

Generalized Anxiety Disorder (GAD):

GAD is characterized by excessive and persistent worry about various aspects of life, such as work, health, or everyday situations. Individuals with GAD often struggle with controlling their worry, leading to significant distress and impairment in daily functioning.

Panic Disorder:

Panic disorder involves recurrent and unexpected panic attacks, which are intense periods of fear or discomfort accompanied by physical symptoms like rapid heartbeat, shortness of breath, and a sense of impending doom. Panic attacks can be debilitating and may lead to a fear of future attacks, impacting one's quality of life.

Social Anxiety Disorder:

Social anxiety disorder is characterized by an intense fear of being judged, embarrassed, or humiliated in social situations. Individuals with social anxiety may avoid social interactions, leading to feelings of isolation and hindering personal and professional growth.

Specific Phobias:

Specific phobias involve an intense and irrational fear of specific objects or situations, such as heights, spiders, or flying. The fear is excessive and can lead to avoidance behaviors, causing disruption in daily life.

Chapter 3: Benefits and Limitations of AI in Anxiety Relief

Title: The Mind-Body Connection

Subtitle: Exploring the Link

Anxiety not only affects the mind but also has a profound impact on the body. Understanding the mind-body connection is crucial for managing anxiety effectively.

Psychological Impact:

Anxiety can generate a constant state of worry and fear, leading to heightened stress levels and emotional distress. It can affect self-esteem, confidence, and overall mental well-being. Recognizing and addressing the psychological impact of anxiety is a vital step towards healing.

Physical Manifestations:

Anxiety often manifests physically, with symptoms such as increased heart rate, shallow breathing, muscle tension, headaches, and digestive issues. These physical manifestations can further exacerbate anxiety, creating a cycle of distress. Learning to manage these physical symptoms is essential for overall anxiety relief.

Cognitive Patterns:

Anxiety can also influence cognitive patterns, leading to negative thinking, excessive self-criticism, and distorted perceptions. Recognizing and challenging these cognitive patterns is an important aspect of anxiety management.

Chapter 4: Getting Started: Setting Up Your AI Tools and Resources

Title: Exploring the Role of AI in Anxiety Management

Subtitle: Harnessing Technology for Support

Artificial Intelligence (AI) has emerged as a powerful tool in various fields, including mental health. In recent years, AI has shown great promise in assisting individuals with anxiety management. In this chapter, we will explore the role of AI in anxiety management and how it can provide valuable support on your journey towards relief.

Understanding AI's Potential:

AI technology has the ability to analyze vast amounts of data, identify patterns, and provide personalized recommendations. When applied to anxiety management, AI can help individuals gain insights into their triggers, offer coping strategies, and provide a sense of companionship and support.

Enhancing Self-Awareness:

AI tools can assist in enhancing self-awareness by tracking and analyzing various aspects of your mental well-being. By monitoring your mood, sleep patterns, and stress levels, AI can help you identify patterns and recognize the factors that contribute to your anxiety. This self-awareness is crucial for developing effective coping mechanisms.

Tailored Recommendations:

One of the significant advantages of AI is its ability to provide personalized recommendations. Based on the data it gathers, AI can suggest specific relaxation techniques, breathing exercises, or activities that may alleviate your anxiety. These tailored recommendations can be invaluable in finding strategies that work best for you.

Accessible Support:

AI-based anxiety management tools offer accessible support that can be accessed anytime and anywhere. Whether through mobile apps, virtual assistants, or online platforms, AI provides a convenient and readily available source of guidance, resources, and coping strategies. This accessibility ensures that support is just a few taps away whenever you need it.

Ethical Considerations:

While AI offers great potential, it is essential to consider the ethical implications. Privacy and data security should be prioritized when using AI tools. Ensure that the platforms you choose adhere to strict privacy standards and protect your personal information.

By exploring the role of AI in anxiety management, you can harness the potential of this technology to augment your existing coping strategies and find effective ways to manage your anxiety. In the following chapters, we will delve deeper into specific AI-based tools and techniques that can provide valuable support on your anxiety relief journey.

Subtitle: Embracing the Potential

Getting started with AI tools for anxiety management can feel overwhelming, but with the right guidance, you can harness their potential to empower yourself on your journey towards relief. This chapter will provide you with the necessary steps to set up your AI tools and resources effectively.

Assess Your Needs:

Before diving into the world of AI-based anxiety support, take some time to assess your specific needs and goals. Consider the areas where you need assistance and identify the aspects of anxiety management that are most important to you. This self-reflection will help you make informed decisions while selecting the right tools.

Research and Explore:

The realm of AI-based anxiety support systems is vast and ever-evolving. Conduct thorough research to explore the available options. Read reviews, compare features, and consider the credibility of the platforms or applications you come across. Look for tools that align with your needs and have a track record of positive user experiences.

Seek Professional Guidance:

While AI tools can be beneficial, it is essential to remember that they are not a substitute for professional help. Consider consulting with a mental health professional who can guide you in integrating AI into your anxiety management plan. They can provide valuable insights and ensure that the tools you choose complement your overall treatment approach.

Chapter 5: Finding the Right AI-Based Anxiety Support Systems

Subtitle: Navigating the Options

AI-based anxiety support systems come in various forms, each offering unique features and approaches to managing anxiety. This chapter will help you navigate the options and find the right support system that suits your needs.

Virtual Assistants:

Virtual assistants, powered by AI, are becoming increasingly popular for anxiety management. These intelligent programs can provide personalized support, offer relaxation techniques, and even engage in conversational therapy. Look for virtual assistants that have a solid foundation in mental health and are designed specifically for anxiety management.

Mobile Applications:

There is a wide range of mobile applications available that leverage AI for anxiety relief. These apps offer features such as guided meditation, breathing exercises, mood tracking, and cognitive behavioral therapy techniques. Consider your preferences and select an app that aligns with your goals and resonates with you personally.

Wearable Devices:

Wearable devices equipped with AI technology can track physiological data and provide real-time feedback on your stress levels. These devices can help you gain insights into your anxiety triggers and assist in managing your symptoms effectively. Look for wearables that are user-friendly, accurate, and integrate seamlessly with other AI-based tools.

Chapter 6: Personalizing Your AI Experience: Tailoring AI Tools to Your Needs

Subtitle: Making it Your Own

To make the most of AI tools for anxiety management, it is crucial to personalize your experience. This chapter will guide you through the process of tailoring AI tools to suit your individual needs.

Customizing Settings:

Explore the customization options available within the AI tools you use. Adjust settings such as voice preference, background sounds, or visual themes to create an environment that promotes relaxation and comfort.

Setting Goals:

Define clear goals for yourself within the AI tools. Whether it's tracking your progress, setting reminders for self-care activities, or establishing targets for practicing relaxation techniques, having specific goals can enhance your engagement and motivation.

Feedback and Iteration:

Pay attention to the feedback provided by the AI tools and make adjustments accordingly. Learn from the insights and suggestions offered by the system and iterate your approach to maximize the benefits. Regularly assess your progress and adapt the tools to meet your evolving needs.

Chapter 7: AI-Powered Relaxation Techniques: Unwinding with Virtual Assistance

Subtitle: Finding Calm in the Digital Age

Incorporating AI-powered relaxation techniques into your anxiety management routine can be a game-changer. This chapter will explore how virtual assistance can help you find calm and relaxation in the digital age.

Guided Meditation:

AI-powered virtual assistants can provide guided meditation sessions tailored to your specific needs. Through soothing voices, calming music, and step-by-step instructions, these virtual assistants can lead you through mindfulness exercises that promote relaxation and reduce anxiety. Whether you prefer short sessions or longer ones, virtual assistance can be a valuable companion on your meditation journey.

Breathing Exercises:

Deep breathing exercises have long been recognized as effective techniques for anxiety reduction. AI-powered virtual assistants can guide you through various breathing exercises, helping you regulate your breath and activate the body's relaxation response. These exercises can be customized to your preferred pace and duration, allowing you to find a rhythm that works best for you.

Progressive Muscle Relaxation:

Progressive muscle relaxation is a technique that involves systematically tensing and releasing different muscle groups to promote relaxation. AI-powered virtual assistants can provide audio instructions and guide you through this process, helping you release tension and achieve a state of deep relaxation. By regularly practicing progressive muscle relaxation, you can reduce muscle tension, alleviate anxiety symptoms, and promote overall well-being.

Mindfulness Practices:

Practicing mindfulness can significantly contribute to anxiety management. AI-powered virtual assistants can offer mindfulness exercises that help you cultivate present-moment awareness, non-judgmental observation, and acceptance. From body scans to mindful walking, these practices can anchor you in the present and reduce anxiety by shifting your focus away from worries and into the present experience.

By incorporating AI-powered relaxation techniques into your daily routine, you can create a dedicated space for calm and rejuvenation. Virtual assistants provide a convenient and accessible way to engage in these practices, allowing you to unwind and find peace in the midst of the digital age.

As we continue further in this book, we will explore additional AI-powered techniques and strategies that can enhance your anxiety management journey. Remember, finding calm is within your reach, and with the assistance of AI, you can develop effective tools to navigate through anxiety and cultivate a greater sense of well-being.

Chapter 8: Cognitive Behavioral Therapy (CBT) with AI: Rewiring Your Thoughts

Cognitive Behavioral Therapy (CBT) is a widely recognized and effective approach for treating anxiety. It focuses on identifying and challenging negative thought patterns and replacing them with more positive and realistic thoughts. When combined with AI, CBT can be even more powerful in helping individuals rewire their thoughts and manage anxiety.

AI-powered tools and applications can assist individuals in CBT by providing personalized feedback, reminders, and resources. For example, an AI chatbot can act as a virtual therapist, guiding individuals through CBT exercises and offering support and encouragement. These chatbots can also track progress and provide insights into patterns of negative thinking, helping individuals identify triggers and develop strategies to challenge and reframe their thoughts.

Furthermore, AI can enhance CBT by providing real-time monitoring and analysis of physiological data, such as heart rate and skin conductance. By integrating AI with wearable devices or smartphone sensors, individuals can gain a deeper understanding of the connection between their thoughts, emotions, and physical responses. This information can then be used to tailor CBT interventions to specific situations or triggers.

In this chapter, we will explore different AI-powered tools and techniques that can support CBT. We will discuss the benefits and limitations of using AI in CBT and provide practical tips for incorporating AI into your anxiety management routine. Additionally, we will address ethical considerations and privacy concerns related to using AI in therapy.

By combining the principles of CBT with the capabilities of AI, individuals can gain valuable insights, receive personalized support, and effectively rewire their thoughts to manage anxiety more effectively.

Chapter 9: Identifying Anxiety Triggers: AI Insights for Self-Awareness

Understanding the triggers that contribute to anxiety is a crucial step in managing and overcoming it. In this chapter, we will explore how AI can provide valuable insights for identifying anxiety triggers and promoting self-awareness.

AI algorithms have the capability to analyze vast amounts of data, including behavioral patterns, physiological responses, and even textual data from social media or personal journals. By leveraging this data, AI can help individuals gain a deeper understanding of their anxiety triggers and patterns.

One way AI can assist in identifying anxiety triggers is through the analysis of behavioral patterns. AI-powered applications can track and analyze various aspects of an individual's behavior, such as sleep patterns, exercise routines, social interactions, and daily activities. By correlating these behaviors with anxiety symptoms, AI can provide insights into specific triggers that may contribute to anxiety.

For example, AI might identify that certain social situations or lack of physical activity are associated with increased anxiety levels.

Another approach is the analysis of physiological responses. AI can monitor and analyze data from wearable devices, such as heart rate monitors or skin conductance sensors, to detect physiological changes associated with anxiety. By identifying specific physiological markers, AI can provide individuals with real-time feedback on their anxiety levels and help them recognize triggers that may cause heightened anxiety responses.

Furthermore, AI can analyze textual data, such as social media posts or personal journals, to identify patterns and themes related to anxiety triggers. Natural Language Processing (NLP) algorithms can extract relevant information and identify recurring words or topics that are associated with anxiety. This can help individuals gain insights into their thoughts, emotions, and external factors that contribute to their anxiety.

By utilizing AI insights for self-awareness, individuals can gain a better understanding of their unique anxiety triggers. This knowledge empowers them to develop personalized strategies for managing and avoiding these triggers. It also allows individuals to proactively address potential triggers and take steps to minimize their impact on their well-being.

In this chapter, we will explore different AI-powered tools and techniques for identifying anxiety triggers. We will discuss the benefits and limitations of using AI in self-awareness and provide practical tips for leveraging AI insights to manage anxiety effectively. Additionally, we will address concerns related to privacy and data security when utilizing AI for self-awareness.

By harnessing the power of AI, individuals can gain valuable insights into their anxiety triggers, leading to a greater sense of self-awareness and improved anxiety management.

Chapter 10: AI Chatbots: 24/7 Support for Anxiety Relief

In this digital age, where access to support and resources is crucial, AI chatbots offer a unique and valuable solution for individuals seeking 24/7 support for anxiety relief. In this chapter, we will explore the role of AI chatbots in providing continuous support and assistance to individuals struggling with anxiety.

AI-powered chatbots are virtual assistants equipped with natural language processing capabilities, enabling them to engage in human-like conversations. These chatbots can offer personalized and empathetic support, providing a safe space for individuals to express their feelings and concerns related to anxiety.

One of the key benefits of AI chatbots is their availability at any time of the day or night. Unlike traditional therapy or helplines, AI chatbots are accessible 24/7, allowing individuals to seek support whenever they need it most. This accessibility is particularly beneficial during moments of heightened anxiety or when immediate assistance is required.

AI chatbots can provide a range of anxiety relief strategies and techniques. They can offer evidence-based coping strategies, such as deep breathing exercises, progressive muscle relaxation, or guided imagery. These techniques can help individuals regulate their emotions, reduce anxiety symptoms, and promote relaxation.

Moreover, AI chatbots can act as virtual companions, providing emotional support and encouragement. They can engage in empathetic conversations, actively listening to individuals and validating their experiences. This human-like interaction can help individuals feel understood and less alone in their struggles with anxiety.

AI chatbots can also offer personalized recommendations and resources based on an individual's specific needs and preferences. They can suggest self-help articles, recommend meditation apps, or provide information about local support groups or therapists. This tailored guidance can empower individuals to take proactive steps towards managing their anxiety effectively.

However, it is important to acknowledge the limitations of AI chatbots. While they can provide valuable support, they should not replace traditional therapy or professional help. AI chatbots are best utilized as a complement to existing mental health resources, offering additional support and guidance.

By leveraging the power of AI chatbots, individuals can access continuous support, guidance, and resources for anxiety relief. These virtual companions offer a convenient and accessible means of managing anxiety in the comfort of one's own space and time.

Chapter 11: AI-Enhanced Meditation and Mindfulness Practices

As technology continues to advance, so does its potential to assist in various aspects of our lives. One area where AI has shown promise is in enhancing meditation and mindfulness practices for anxiety sufferers. In this chapter, we will explore the ways in which AI can be utilized to provide personalized and effective support for individuals seeking relief from anxiety.

Understanding the Role of AI in Meditation and Mindfulness:

AI algorithms can analyze vast amounts of data to identify patterns and provide insights into individual anxiety triggers and responses.

Machine learning algorithms can adapt and personalize meditation and mindfulness practices based on an individual's specific needs and preferences.

AI-powered virtual assistants can guide individuals through meditation sessions, offering customized guidance and support.

Personalized Meditation Experiences:

AI algorithms can analyze an individual's physiological responses, such as heart rate and breathing patterns, to tailor meditation practices that are most effective for them.

Virtual reality (VR) and augmented reality (AR) technologies can create immersive environments that promote relaxation and focus during meditation.

AI-powered virtual assistants can provide real-time feedback and suggestions to help individuals deepen their meditation practice.

Mindfulness Training and Anxiety Management:

AI algorithms can help individuals identify and manage anxiety-inducing thoughts and emotions by providing real-time insights and coping strategies.

AI-powered chatbots can offer 24/7 support, allowing individuals to practice mindfulness at any time they need it.

Virtual reality simulations can help individuals confront and overcome anxiety-provoking situations in a controlled and supportive environment.

Tracking Progress and Providing Insights:

AI algorithms can track an individual's meditation and mindfulness practices over time, providing personalized insights into progress and areas for improvement.

Machine learning models can identify correlations between specific meditation techniques and anxiety reduction, helping individuals fine-tune their practice.

AI-powered apps and wearables can provide reminders and encouragement to maintain a consistent meditation routine.

Ethical Considerations and Human Support:

While AI can offer valuable support, it is essential to remember that human connection and support are crucial for anxiety sufferers.

AI should be seen as a complement to, rather than a replacement for, human therapists and support networks.

Privacy and data security should be prioritized when using AI in meditation and mindfulness practices.

In conclusion, AI has the potential to revolutionize meditation and mindfulness practices for anxiety sufferers. By leveraging AI algorithms, virtual reality, and personalized guidance, individuals can access tailored support that adapts to their specific needs. However, it is important to remember that AI should be used in conjunction with human support to ensure a holistic approach to anxiety management.

Chapter 12: Tracking and Analyzing Anxiety Patterns with AI

In the previous chapters, we explored the potential of AI to enhance meditation and mindfulness practices for anxiety sufferers. Now, let's delve into the practical aspects of utilizing AI to track and analyze anxiety patterns. By leveraging AI algorithms and tools, individuals can gain valuable insights into their anxiety triggers, responses, and progress. This chapter will guide you through the process of tracking and analyzing anxiety patterns using AI, providing explanations on what resources to use, how to use them, and why they are beneficial.

AI-Powered Mood and Anxiety Tracking Apps:

Utilize AI-powered mood and anxiety tracking apps to record and monitor your emotional state and anxiety levels throughout the day.

These apps use machine learning algorithms to analyze your input and provide visualizations of your anxiety patterns over time.

By regularly tracking your anxiety, you can identify trends, triggers, and potential correlations between your daily activities and anxiety levels.

Wearable Devices and Biofeedback:

Wearable devices, such as smartwatches or fitness trackers, equipped with sensors can monitor physiological signals like heart rate, sleep patterns, and skin conductance.

Use AI-powered biofeedback tools to analyze the data collected by wearable devices and gain insights into how your body responds to anxiety-inducing situations.

By understanding your physiological responses, you can become more aware of anxiety triggers and develop strategies to manage them effectively.

Natural Language Processing (NLP) for Journaling:

Use AI-powered journaling apps that employ natural language processing (NLP) algorithms to analyze your written entries.

These apps can identify recurring themes, emotions, and patterns in your journal entries, helping you gain deeper insights into your anxiety triggers and thought patterns.

Regular journaling with NLP analysis can assist in identifying patterns that may be difficult to recognize through self-reflection alone.

Machine Learning for Anxiety Prediction:

Explore machine learning models that can predict anxiety episodes based on various input data, such as daily activities, sleep patterns, or physiological signals.

By training these models with your personal data, you can receive alerts or notifications when the likelihood of an anxiety episode is high, allowing you to take proactive measures.

Machine learning algorithms can also identify patterns in your behavior that precede anxiety episodes, helping you understand warning signs and implement preventive strategies.

Personalized Recommendations and Interventions:

AI algorithms can provide personalized recommendations and interventions based on the analysis of your anxiety patterns.

These recommendations may include specific meditation techniques, breathing exercises, or activities that have proven effective in managing your anxiety.

By leveraging AI-powered tools, you can receive tailored suggestions to address your unique anxiety triggers and responses.

Remember, while AI can provide valuable insights and support, it is essential to integrate these tools into a comprehensive anxiety management plan that includes professional help and human support. AI should be seen as a complement to, rather than a replacement for, traditional therapeutic approaches.

In conclusion, tracking and analyzing anxiety patterns with AI can provide individuals with valuable insights into their triggers, responses, and progress. By utilizing AI-powered mood tracking apps, wearable devices, NLP journaling tools, machine learning models, and personalized recommendations, individuals can gain a deeper understanding of their anxiety and develop effective strategies for managing it. Embrace the power of AI as a tool to support your journey towards anxiety relief and well-being.

Chapter 13: AI-Driven Journaling: Expressive Therapy for Anxiety

Journaling has long been recognized as a therapeutic practice for promoting self-reflection and emotional well-being. With the advancements in AI technology, individuals can now leverage AI-driven journaling to enhance their anxiety management journey. In this chapter, we will explore how AI can be used to facilitate expressive therapy for anxiety.

AI-Powered Journaling Apps:

Utilize AI-powered journaling apps that employ natural language processing (NLP) algorithms to analyze your written entries.

These apps can provide insights into your emotions, thought patterns, and recurring themes in your journal entries related to anxiety.

AI-driven journaling can help you gain a deeper understanding of your anxiety triggers, identify patterns, and discover new perspectives.

Emotional Analysis and Sentiment Tracking:

AI algorithms can analyze the emotional tone and sentiment of your journal entries to provide an objective assessment of your emotional state.

By tracking your emotional patterns over time, you can identify triggers and patterns that contribute to anxiety.

AI-driven sentiment analysis can help you recognize and address negative thinking patterns, promoting a more positive and balanced mindset.

Guided Prompts and Reflections:

AI-powered journaling apps can offer guided prompts and reflections tailored to your specific needs and goals.

These prompts can encourage self-reflection, mindfulness, and exploration of emotions related to anxiety.

AI-driven guidance can help you dive deeper into your thoughts and emotions, facilitating a more comprehensive understanding of your anxiety.

Personalized Insights and Recommendations:

AI algorithms can provide personalized insights and recommendations based on the analysis of your journal entries.

These insights may include coping strategies, mindfulness exercises, or suggestions for professional support.

By leveraging AI-driven journaling, you can receive tailored recommendations to support your anxiety management journey.

Chapter 14: AI-Powered Sleep Solutions: Restoring Peaceful Nights

Sleep plays a crucial role in our overall well-being, and anxiety can often disrupt our ability to get a good night's rest. Fortunately, AI can provide innovative solutions to help individuals struggling with anxiety-induced sleep disturbances. In this chapter, we will explore how AI can power sleep solutions to restore peaceful nights.

Sleep Tracking and Analysis:

Utilize AI-powered sleep tracking apps or wearable devices to monitor your sleep patterns, such as duration, quality, and disruptions.

AI algorithms can analyze the data collected and provide insights into your sleep patterns, highlighting potential correlations with anxiety.

By understanding the relationship between anxiety and sleep, you can develop targeted strategies to improve your sleep quality.

AI-Enhanced Relaxation Techniques:

AI-powered apps and devices can offer guided relaxation techniques, such as breathing exercises or soothing sounds, to promote relaxation before bedtime.

These tools can adapt to your specific needs and preferences, providing a personalized experience to help you unwind and prepare for sleep.

AI-driven relaxation techniques can help alleviate anxiety symptoms that often interfere with falling asleep.

Smart Sleep Environment:

AI-powered smart home devices can create a sleep-friendly environment by adjusting lighting, temperature, and noise levels to optimize your sleep conditions.

These devices can also provide soothing sounds or white noise to mask disruptive noises that may trigger anxiety.

By creating a calming and supportive sleep environment, AI can help you establish a bedtime routine that promotes relaxation and restful sleep.

Sleep-Wake Transition Assistance:

AI-powered alarm clocks can wake you up gently during the optimal phase of your sleep cycle, minimizing grogginess and promoting a refreshed start to the day.

These devices can also provide gentle reminders and suggestions for maintaining a consistent sleep schedule.

AI-driven sleep-wake transition assistance can help regulate your sleep patterns and promote a more regular sleep routine.

By leveraging AI-powered sleep solutions, individuals can address anxiety-related sleep disturbances and restore peaceful nights. The combination of AI-driven sleep tracking, personalized relaxation techniques, a smart sleep environment, and sleep-wake transition assistance can significantly improve your sleep quality and overall well-being.

Sleep Recommendations and Insights:

  - AI algorithms can analyze your sleep data and provide personalized recommendations to improve your sleep hygiene and address anxiety-related sleep disturbances.

  - These recommendations may include adjustments to your bedtime routine, suggestions for creating a sleep-friendly environment, or strategies to manage anxiety before sleep.

  - By following AI-driven insights and recommendations, you can establish healthy sleep habits that support better sleep and reduce anxiety.

Sleep Coaching and Support:

  - AI-powered sleep solutions can offer virtual sleep coaching and support, guiding you through the process of improving your sleep habits and managing anxiety-related sleep issues.

  - Virtual sleep coaches can provide educational resources, personalized guidance, and motivation to help you stay on track with your sleep goals.

  - AI-driven sleep coaching can empower you with the knowledge and tools to overcome sleep challenges and achieve restful nights.

Remember, while AI-powered sleep solutions can be beneficial, it is important to complement them with other healthy sleep practices and seek professional help if needed. AI should be seen as a tool to support your sleep journey, but not a substitute for medical advice or treatment.

In conclusion, AI-powered sleep solutions offer innovative approaches to address anxiety-related sleep disturbances and restore peaceful nights. By leveraging AI-driven sleep tracking, relaxation techniques, smart sleep environments, sleep-wake transition assistance, personalized recommendations, and virtual sleep coaching, individuals can improve their sleep quality, manage anxiety, and promote overall well-being. Embrace the power of AI to transform your sleep and wake up feeling refreshed and rejuvenated.

Chapter 15: Virtual Reality (VR) and Augmented Reality (AR) for Anxiety Management

Virtual Reality (VR) and Augmented Reality (AR) technologies have shown great potential in various fields, including anxiety management. In this chapter, we will explore how VR and AR can be utilized to create immersive experiences that help individuals effectively manage their anxiety.

Exposure Therapy in Virtual Environments:

VR technology can create realistic simulations of anxiety-inducing situations in a controlled and safe environment.

Individuals can gradually expose themselves to these virtual scenarios, allowing them to confront and overcome their fears and anxieties.

VR exposure therapy has been proven to be an effective treatment for various anxiety disorders, such as phobias and social anxiety.

Mindfulness and Relaxation in Virtual Environments:

VR and AR can transport individuals to serene and peaceful virtual environments, promoting relaxation and mindfulness.

By immersing oneself in these calming virtual spaces, individuals can reduce stress, anxiety, and promote a sense of tranquility.

Guided meditation and mindfulness exercises can be enhanced through VR and AR, providing a more immersive and engaging experience.

Skills Training and Cognitive Behavioral Therapy:

VR and AR can be used to simulate real-life scenarios that are challenging for individuals with anxiety.

Through these simulations, individuals can practice and develop coping skills, such as assertiveness or problem-solving techniques.

Cognitive behavioral therapy techniques can be integrated into VR and AR experiences, helping individuals reframe negative thoughts and behaviors.

Biofeedback Integration:

VR and AR technologies can be combined with biofeedback devices to provide real-time physiological feedback during anxiety management sessions.

Individuals can monitor their heart rate, breathing patterns, or skin conductance responses, helping them become more aware of their anxiety symptoms.

Biofeedback integration in VR and AR can assist individuals in learning self-regulation techniques to manage and reduce anxiety symptoms.

Chapter 16: AI-Enabled Biofeedback: Monitoring and Regulating Anxiety Symptoms

Biofeedback is a technique that allows individuals to monitor and regulate their physiological responses to better manage anxiety symptoms. With the help of AI, biofeedback becomes even more powerful in providing personalized support. In this chapter, we will explore how AI-enabled biofeedback can help individuals monitor and regulate their anxiety symptoms effectively.

Wearable Devices and Sensors:

Wearable devices equipped with sensors can track physiological signals, such as heart rate, skin conductance, or breathing patterns.

AI algorithms can analyze the data collected by these devices, providing insights into an individual's anxiety symptoms and triggers.

Wearable devices can also provide real-time feedback and alerts to help individuals recognize and manage their anxiety symptoms.

Personalized Biofeedback Training:

AI algorithms can adapt biofeedback training programs to an individual's specific needs and responses.

By analyzing the collected data, AI can provide personalized recommendations and techniques to help individuals regulate their anxiety symptoms effectively.

AI-enabled biofeedback training can empower individuals with the tools and strategies to manage their anxiety in real-time.

Mobile Apps for Biofeedback:

AI-powered mobile apps can transform smartphones into biofeedback devices, allowing individuals to monitor their anxiety symptoms on the go.

These apps can provide real-time visualizations and feedback based on an individual's physiological responses.

By using AI-enabled biofeedback apps, individuals can develop self-awareness and gain control over their anxiety symptoms wherever they are.

Integration with Therapy and Treatment:

AI-enabled biofeedback can complement traditional therapy approaches by providing objective data and insights into an individual's anxiety symptoms.

Therapists can utilize the information gathered through AI-enabled biofeedback to tailor treatment plans and monitor progress.

AI can assist in identifying patterns and trends in an individual's anxiety symptoms, helping therapists make informed decisions about treatment interventions.

By leveraging VR, AR, and AI-enabled biofeedback techniques, therapists can create immersive and personalized experiences for individuals with anxiety disorders. Virtual reality simulations can expose individuals to anxiety-inducing situations in a controlled environment, allowing them to practice coping strategies and gradually desensitize themselves to triggers.

AI algorithms can analyze the physiological responses and behaviors observed during these virtual reality sessions, providing therapists with valuable insights into an individual's progress and areas that require further attention. This data-driven approach enables therapists to tailor treatment plans and interventions to each individual's specific needs.

Furthermore, AI-enabled biofeedback can also be integrated with other treatment modalities, such as medication management. By monitoring an individual's physiological responses and anxiety symptoms in real-time, AI algorithms can assist in optimizing medication dosages and schedules, ensuring that individuals receive the most effective and personalized treatment.

In conclusion, AI-enabled biofeedback holds immense potential in monitoring and regulating anxiety symptoms. By leveraging wearable devices, mobile apps, and integration with therapy and treatment, individuals can receive personalized support, gain self-awareness, and develop effective strategies to manage their anxiety in real-time. The combination of AI and biofeedback has the power to revolutionize anxiety management and improve the overall well-being of individuals.

Chapter 17: Ethical Considerations in AI-Based Anxiety Support

As AI technology continues to advance and play a significant role in anxiety support, it is crucial to address the ethical considerations associated with its implementation. In this chapter, we will explore some key ethical considerations that arise when using AI for anxiety support.

Privacy and Data Security:

AI-based anxiety support systems rely on collecting and analyzing personal data to provide personalized recommendations. It is essential to ensure that individuals' privacy is protected and their data is securely stored and used only for the intended purpose. Transparent data practices, informed consent, and robust security measures should be in place to safeguard sensitive information.

Bias and Fairness:

AI algorithms are trained on large datasets, which may contain biases that can perpetuate existing inequalities. It is crucial to address bias in the development and deployment of AI-based anxiety support systems to ensure fairness and equal access for all individuals. Regular audits and ongoing monitoring can help identify and mitigate biases in the algorithms.

Informed Consent and Autonomy:

Individuals should have the right to understand how AI-based anxiety support systems work and the potential risks and benefits associated with their use. Informed consent should be obtained, and individuals should have the autonomy to choose whether they want to engage with these systems or opt-out at any time. Clear and understandable explanations of how the AI algorithms work should be provided.

Human Oversight and Accountability:

While AI can provide valuable support in managing anxiety, it is crucial to maintain human oversight and accountability. Professionals, such as therapists or healthcare providers, should be involved in the development and monitoring of AI-based systems to ensure that the technology is used appropriately and in alignment with ethical standards. Regular evaluations and audits can help identify and address any potential issues.

Transparency and Explainability:

AI algorithms can be complex and difficult to understand. It is important to ensure transparency and explainability in the functioning of AI-based anxiety support systems. Individuals should have access to understandable explanations of how the algorithms make recommendations and decisions. This transparency can help build trust and enable individuals to make informed choices about their anxiety support.

Continual Evaluation and Improvement:

AI-based anxiety support systems should undergo continual evaluation and improvement to ensure their effectiveness and ethical use. Regular assessments of the system's performance, impact, and potential unintended consequences should be conducted. Feedback from individuals using the system should be actively sought and incorporated into the system's development and improvement processes.

In conclusion, as AI-based anxiety support systems become more prevalent, it is essential to address the ethical considerations associated with their use. Privacy, bias, informed consent, human oversight, transparency, and continual evaluation are key areas that require attention. By addressing these ethical considerations, we can ensure that AI-based anxiety support systems are developed and used in a responsible and ethical manner, ultimately benefiting individuals in their journey towards managing anxiety.

Chapter 18: Integrating Human Connection with AI Support Systems

While AI support systems have proven to be valuable tools in managing anxiety, it is essential to recognize the importance of human connection in providing comprehensive support. In this chapter, we will explore the significance of integrating human connection with AI support systems for anxiety management.

Emotional Support and Empathy:

AI support systems can provide personalized recommendations and strategies, but they may lack the ability to offer emotional support and empathy that humans can provide. Human connection plays a crucial role in creating a safe and understanding environment for individuals with anxiety. Professionals, such as therapists or support groups, can offer empathy, active listening, and emotional guidance that can complement the AI-based support.

Individualized Care and Flexibility:

AI support systems excel in providing personalized recommendations based on data analysis. However, human connection allows for individualized care that takes into account contextual factors, personal experiences, and unique needs. Professionals can adapt their approaches, therapies, and interventions to cater to the specific requirements of each individual, providing a level of flexibility that AI systems may not be able to achieve.

Trust and Relationship Building:

Building a trusting relationship is crucial in anxiety management. While AI systems can provide valuable insights and recommendations, trust is often built through human interaction. Professionals can establish trust by actively listening, understanding individual concerns, and working collaboratively towards managing anxiety. This trust can enhance the effectiveness of the overall support system.

Complex Problem-Solving and Critical Thinking:

Anxiety management often involves complex problem-solving and critical thinking. While AI systems can offer recommendations, human professionals possess the ability to analyze complex situations, identify underlying issues, and guide individuals through the decision-making process. Their expertise and experience contribute to a holistic approach in anxiety management.

Ethical Decision-Making and Accountability:

Human professionals are bound by ethical guidelines and professional codes of conduct, ensuring that they act in the best interests of the individuals they support. They can navigate complex ethical dilemmas and provide guidance on important decisions. Integrating human connection with AI support systems ensures ethical decision-making and accountability in anxiety management.

Continuity and Long-Term Support:

Human connection provides continuity and long-term support in anxiety management. Professionals can establish ongoing relationships with individuals, monitoring progress, adjusting interventions, and providing support throughout their journey. This continuous support is essential for maintaining progress and preventing relapse.

In conclusion, while AI support systems offer valuable tools for managing anxiety, integrating human connection is crucial for comprehensive support. Emotional support, individualized care, trust-building, complex problem-solving, ethical decision-making, and continuity are all aspects that human professionals bring to the table. By combining the strengths of AI systems with human connection, we can create a holistic and effective support system that addresses the multifaceted nature of anxiety management.

Chapter 19: Combining Traditional and AI Approaches for Holistic Anxiety Relief

In the quest for holistic anxiety relief, it is valuable to combine traditional approaches with AI technology to create comprehensive and effective support systems. In this chapter, we will explore the benefits of integrating traditional and AI approaches in managing anxiety.

Personalized Treatment Plans:

Traditional approaches, such as therapy and counseling, offer individualized care based on face-to-face interactions. By incorporating AI technology, personalized treatment plans can be enhanced with data-driven insights. AI algorithms can analyze vast amounts of data to identify patterns, triggers, and effective strategies, providing therapists with valuable information to tailor treatment plans to each individual's specific needs.

Enhanced Self-Awareness:

Traditional approaches often focus on developing self-awareness and understanding one's thoughts, emotions, and behaviors. AI technology can complement these efforts by providing real-time feedback and data visualization. Individuals can track their anxiety symptoms, physiological responses, and progress over time, gaining deeper insights into their triggers and patterns. This enhanced self-awareness empowers individuals to make informed decisions and take proactive steps in managing their anxiety.

Accessible Support:

One of the significant advantages of AI technology is its accessibility. AI-powered mobile apps, chatbots, and virtual support systems can provide round-the-clock assistance, making support readily available whenever individuals need it. This accessibility ensures that individuals have continuous access to resources and strategies to manage their anxiety, even outside of traditional therapy sessions.

Targeted Intervention:

Combining traditional and AI approaches allows for targeted intervention. Traditional therapy sessions can address deep-rooted issues, provide emotional support, and offer guidance in complex situations. AI technology, on the other hand, can provide real-time feedback, reminders, and coping strategies in everyday life. This combination ensures that individuals receive comprehensive support tailored to their unique needs, both in and outside of therapy sessions.

Long-Term Progress Monitoring:

Traditional approaches often involve periodic therapy sessions, making it challenging to monitor progress consistently. AI technology can bridge this gap by continuously collecting and analyzing data, providing therapists with objective insights into an individual's progress. This real-time monitoring enables therapists to make informed decisions, adjust treatment plans, and intervene when necessary, ensuring long-term progress and preventing relapse.

Collaborative Approach:

Integrating traditional and AI approaches encourages a collaborative approach between individuals and their healthcare professionals. Therapists can incorporate AI technology as a tool in therapy sessions, guiding individuals in utilizing AI-powered resources effectively. This collaboration fosters a sense of empowerment and active participation in the anxiety management process.

In conclusion, combining traditional and AI approaches for anxiety relief offers a holistic and comprehensive support system. Personalized treatment plans, enhanced self-awareness, accessible support, targeted intervention, long-term progress monitoring, and a collaborative approach are some of the benefits of integrating these approaches. By leveraging the strengths of both traditional and AI methods, individuals can receive tailored, accessible, and effective support in managing their anxiety, ultimately leading to improved overall well-being.

Chapter 20: AI and Professional Therapy: Collaborative Care for Anxiety

In the field of anxiety management, the integration of AI technology with professional therapy can create a powerful collaborative care approach. This chapter explores the benefits and potential of combining AI and professional therapy for comprehensive anxiety care.

Augmented Assessment:

AI technology can assist therapists in the assessment process by analyzing large amounts of data and identifying patterns in an individual's anxiety symptoms. By integrating AI-powered assessment tools, therapists can gain deeper insights into an individual's condition, enabling more accurate diagnoses and personalized treatment plans. This augmented assessment enhances the effectiveness and efficiency of the therapeutic process.

Data-Driven Insights:

AI algorithms can analyze data collected through various sources, such as wearable devices, mobile apps, and online platforms. These insights provide therapists with objective information about an individual's anxiety symptoms, triggers, and progress. By incorporating these data-driven insights into therapy sessions, therapists can tailor interventions and strategies to address specific needs, ultimately improving the outcomes of therapy.

Personalized Treatment Plans:

AI technology can contribute to the development of personalized treatment plans by leveraging data analysis. By considering an individual's unique characteristics, preferences, and responses, AI algorithms can recommend specific interventions, coping strategies, and therapeutic techniques. This personalized approach ensures that therapy aligns closely with an individual's needs, enhancing the effectiveness of the treatment.

Continuous Support:

While therapy sessions are typically scheduled at regular intervals, anxiety symptoms can arise at any time. AI-powered tools, such as mobile apps or chatbots, can provide continuous support outside of therapy sessions. These tools can offer real-time coping strategies, reminders, and resources to help individuals manage their anxiety in everyday life. The combination of professional therapy and AI-based support ensures that individuals have access to assistance whenever they need it.

Remote Therapy and Telehealth:

AI technology enables remote therapy and telehealth options, which can be particularly beneficial for individuals who face barriers to in-person therapy, such as geographical distance or physical limitations. Through video conferencing, online platforms, and AI-powered tools, therapists can provide therapy sessions and support remotely, ensuring that individuals receive necessary care regardless of their location.

Therapist-Client Collaboration:

The integration of AI technology does not replace the role of therapists; rather, it enhances their capabilities. Therapists can collaborate with AI systems to provide a more comprehensive and tailored approach to anxiety care. They can interpret AI-generated insights, validate recommendations, and adapt interventions based on their clinical expertise. This collaboration ensures that therapy remains a human-centered process while leveraging the benefits of AI technology.

In conclusion, the collaboration between AI technology and professional therapy offers a promising approach to anxiety care.

Augmented assessment, data-driven insights, personalized treatment plans, continuous support, remote therapy options, and therapist-client collaboration are key benefits of this collaborative care model. By harnessing the strengths of both AI and professional therapy, individuals can receive comprehensive, personalized, and accessible care for managing their anxiety, leading to improved well-being and long-term success.

Chapter 21: Overcoming Stigma: Addressing Concerns about AI-Based Support

While AI-based support systems have the potential to revolutionize anxiety management, it is essential to address concerns and overcome the stigma associated with relying on AI for support. In this chapter, we will explore common concerns and provide insights on how to address them.

1. Fear of Replacement:

One concern individuals may have is the fear that AI-based support systems will replace human professionals. It is crucial to emphasize that AI is meant to augment and enhance, rather than replace, human support. AI technology can provide valuable tools, insights, and resources, but the human connection and expertise of professionals remain integral to the support process.

2. Lack of Personalization:

Some individuals may worry that AI-based support systems lack personalization and may not understand their unique experiences. It is important to highlight that AI technology can be tailored to individual needs through data analysis and algorithms. AI systems can adapt and provide personalized recommendations based on an individual's specific symptoms, triggers, and progress, ensuring a personalized approach to anxiety management.

3. Privacy and Data Security:

Privacy and data security are valid concerns when using AI-based support systems. It is crucial to address these concerns by implementing robust security measures, transparent data practices, and obtaining informed consent. Clear communication about how data is collected, stored, and used can help alleviate concerns and build trust in the use of AI technology for anxiety support.

4. Ethical Considerations:

Ethical considerations, such as bias, accountability, and transparency, are important when implementing AI-based support systems. It is essential to prioritize ethical guidelines, regularly evaluate and address biases, involve human oversight in the development and monitoring of AI systems, and ensure transparency in how AI algorithms make recommendations and decisions. By addressing these ethical considerations, individuals can feel more confident in utilizing AI-based support.

5. Integration with Human Connection:

To overcome concerns about the lack of human connection, it is crucial to emphasize that AI technology is meant to complement, not replace, human support. Highlight the benefits of integrating AI with professional therapy, emphasizing the collaborative approach that combines the strengths of both AI and human professionals. This integration ensures that individuals receive comprehensive and holistic support that includes empathy, emotional guidance, and complex problem-solving.

6. Education and Awareness:

Education and awareness play a vital role in overcoming stigma and concerns about AI-based support. Provide clear and accessible information about the benefits, limitations, and ethical considerations of AI technology in anxiety management. Foster open discussions, address concerns, and highlight success stories to demonstrate the positive impact of AI-based support systems.

In conclusion, addressing concerns and overcoming stigma surrounding AI-based support systems requires clear communication, emphasizing the collaborative nature of AI and human support, prioritizing privacy and ethical considerations, and fostering education and awareness. By addressing these concerns, individuals can embrace and benefit from the potential of AI technology in managing anxiety, ultimately improving their overall well-being.

Chapter 22: Evaluating the Effectiveness of AI Tools for Anxiety Relief

Introduction:

As the use of artificial intelligence (AI) tools for anxiety relief continues to grow, it is important to evaluate their effectiveness. This chapter explores the various methods used to assess the impact of AI tools on anxiety and provides insights into the evaluation process.

Research Design:

To evaluate the effectiveness of AI tools for anxiety relief, researchers employ different research designs. Randomized controlled trials (RCTs) are commonly used, where participants are randomly assigned to receive either the AI intervention or a control condition. Other designs, such as pre-post studies and observational studies, are also utilized to gather valuable data.

Outcome Measures:

To measure the effectiveness of AI tools, researchers use various outcome measures. Self-report questionnaires, such as the State-Trait Anxiety Inventory (STAI) and the Generalized Anxiety Disorder-7

(GAD-7), are commonly used to assess anxiety levels. Additionally, physiological measures like heart rate variability and skin conductance can provide objective data on anxiety reduction.

User Experience:

Evaluating the user experience is crucial to understanding the effectiveness of AI tools for anxiety relief. Qualitative methods, such as interviews and focus groups, help gather insights into users' perceptions, satisfaction, and overall experience with the AI intervention.

Long-Term Effects:

Assessing the long-term effects of AI tools for anxiety relief is essential. Longitudinal studies can provide valuable information about the sustainability of anxiety reduction and the potential for relapse after using AI tools. Follow-up assessments conducted weeks or months after the intervention can shed light on the lasting impact of AI tools.

Comparative Studies:

Comparative studies comparing AI tools to traditional anxiety relief interventions, such as therapy or medication, can provide valuable insights into the effectiveness of AI tools. These studies help determine whether AI tools are as effective as or even more effective than traditional approaches.

Ethical Considerations:

Evaluating the effectiveness of AI tools for anxiety relief also involves considering ethical implications. Researchers must ensure participant safety, privacy, and informed consent throughout the evaluation process. Transparency in data collection, algorithmic decision-making, and potential biases is crucial.

Conclusion:

Evaluating the effectiveness of AI tools for anxiety relief is a complex process that requires careful consideration of research design, outcome measures, user experience, long-term effects, comparative studies, and ethical considerations. By utilizing a comprehensive evaluation approach, researchers can provide valuable insights into the impact of AI tools on anxiety relief.

Chapter 23: Navigating Privacy and Security in AI-Driven Solutions for Anxiety Sufferers

Introduction:

As anxiety sufferers turn to AI-driven solutions for support, it is crucial to consider their unique needs and the care they should take when using these tools. This chapter explores the key considerations and strategies for anxiety sufferers to navigate privacy and security in AI-driven solutions.

Protecting Personal Information:

Anxiety sufferers should prioritize protecting their personal information when using AI-driven solutions. This involves being cautious about the type and amount of personal data shared with AI tools. It is essential to read and understand the privacy policies and terms of service of AI applications to ensure the responsible handling of personal information.

Choosing Trusted and Secure AI Tools:

Anxiety sufferers should carefully select AI tools that prioritize privacy and security. Researching and choosing reputable and well-established AI applications can help ensure the protection of personal data. Reading user reviews and looking for certifications or endorsements from trusted sources can assist in making informed decisions.

Understanding Data Handling Practices:

Anxiety sufferers should have a clear understanding of how AI tools handle their data. It is important to know what data is collected, how it is stored and transmitted, and who has access to it. Choosing AI tools that are transparent about their data handling practices can help anxiety sufferers make informed choices.

Opting for Anonymity:

Some anxiety sufferers may prefer to maintain anonymity when using AI-driven solutions. It is important to check if AI tools offer options to use the service without revealing personal information. Anonymity can provide an added layer of privacy and help anxiety sufferers feel more comfortable using AI tools.

Monitoring for Potential Risks:

Anxiety sufferers should actively monitor for potential privacy and security risks when using AI-driven solutions. This includes regularly reviewing privacy settings, checking for updates or patches, and being cautious about sharing personal information in public forums or chatbots. Staying informed about potential risks can help maintain privacy and security.

Seeking Professional Guidance:

Anxiety sufferers should consider seeking professional guidance when using AI-driven solutions. Mental health professionals can provide valuable insights and recommendations on using AI tools effectively and safely. They can also help individuals navigate privacy and security concerns specific to their anxiety management journey.

Conclusion:

For anxiety sufferers, navigating privacy and security in AI-driven solutions requires specific considerations and care. By prioritizing the protection of personal information, choosing trusted and secure AI tools, understanding data handling practices, opting for anonymity when desired, monitoring for risks, and seeking professional guidance, anxiety sufferers can use AI tools to support their mental health journey while maintaining privacy and security.

Chapter 24: AI and Self-Care: Integrating Healthy Habits into Your Routine for Anxiety Sufferers

Introduction:

For anxiety sufferers, incorporating AI into self-care routines can be particularly beneficial. This chapter explores how AI can be utilized to support anxiety management and promote healthy habits for individuals dealing with anxiety.

Personalized Anxiety Management:

AI-powered applications can offer personalized anxiety management recommendations tailored to the specific needs of anxiety sufferers. These recommendations may include techniques for relaxation, grounding exercises, cognitive behavioral therapy (CBT) strategies, and exposure therapy exercises. AI can adapt to individual preferences and provide guidance on managing anxiety symptoms effectively.

Anxiety Tracking and Coping Reminders:

AI tools can assist anxiety sufferers in tracking their anxiety levels and provide reminders for implementing coping strategies. By monitoring anxiety symptoms and offering timely reminders for deep breathing exercises, mindfulness practices, or seeking support, individuals can better manage their anxiety throughout the day.

Cognitive Distortion Identification:

AI algorithms can help anxiety sufferers identify and challenge cognitive distortions, which are common thought patterns associated with anxiety. By analyzing language patterns and providing feedback, AI tools can assist individuals in recognizing and reframing negative thoughts, promoting more positive and realistic thinking.

Virtual Support and Peer Communities:

AI-driven platforms can connect anxiety sufferers with virtual support networks and peer communities. These platforms allow individuals to share experiences, provide support, and access resources specific to anxiety management. AI can facilitate these connections and provide a sense of community for anxiety sufferers.

Sleep and Anxiety Management:

AI can assist anxiety sufferers in improving sleep hygiene, which is crucial for managing anxiety. AI-powered sleep trackers can monitor sleep patterns, provide insights on sleep quality, and offer recommendations for optimizing sleep routines. By addressing sleep disturbances, anxiety sufferers can experience improved overall well-being.

Ethical Considerations:

When utilizing AI for anxiety self-care, ethical considerations remain important. Anxiety sufferers should prioritize the privacy and security of their personal data. It is essential to choose AI applications that uphold strict data protection measures and comply with relevant privacy regulations.

Conclusion:

By integrating AI into self-care routines, anxiety sufferers can enhance their anxiety management strategies, promote healthy habits, and improve overall well-being. Personalized anxiety management, tracking and coping reminders, cognitive distortion identification, virtual support networks, sleep optimization, and ethical considerations are key aspects to consider when incorporating AI into self-care practices for anxiety management.

Chapter 25: AI-Powered Anxiety Apps: A Comprehensive Review

Introduction:

AI-powered anxiety apps have gained popularity as tools to support anxiety management. This chapter provides a comprehensive review of various AI-powered anxiety apps, evaluating their features, effectiveness, user experience, and potential benefits for anxiety sufferers.

1. App Features and Functionality:

The review examines the features and functionality of AI-powered anxiety apps. This includes analyzing the AI algorithms used, the types of anxiety management techniques offered (such as cognitive behavioral therapy, mindfulness exercises, or relaxation techniques), and any unique features that set the apps apart.

2. Effectiveness and Evidence-Based Approaches:

The review assesses the effectiveness of AI-powered anxiety apps by examining the available research and evidence supporting their impact on anxiety management. It considers studies that evaluate the apps' ability to reduce anxiety symptoms, improve well-being, and enhance coping mechanisms. The review also looks for adherence to evidence-based approaches in the app's design and content.

3. User Experience and Interface:

The review evaluates the user experience and interface of AI-powered anxiety apps. It considers factors such as ease of use, visual design, intuitiveness, customization options, and accessibility features. User feedback and ratings are also taken into account to assess the overall user satisfaction and engagement with the app.

4. Privacy and Security:

The review examines the privacy and security measures implemented by AI-powered anxiety apps. It assesses how the apps handle user data, whether they employ encryption and secure storage practices, and if they comply with relevant privacy regulations. Transparency in data usage and the app's privacy policy are also considered.

5. Integration with Other Tools and Support:

The review explores whether AI-powered anxiety apps integrate with other tools or support systems. This includes compatibility with wearable devices, integration with electronic health records, and the availability of additional support resources such as virtual therapy sessions or access to mental health professionals.

6. Cost and Accessibility:

The review considers the cost and accessibility of AI-powered anxiety apps. It examines whether the apps are free or require a subscription, and if there are options for in-app purchases. The availability of the app on multiple platforms (such as iOS and Android) and in different languages is also taken into account.

Conclusion:

The comprehensive review of AI-powered anxiety apps provides valuable insights into their features, effectiveness, user experience, privacy and security measures, integration with other tools and support systems, cost, and accessibility. By considering these factors, anxiety sufferers can make informed decisions about which AI-powered anxiety app may best suit their needs and support their anxiety management journey.

Here are some popular AI-powered anxiety apps along with their platforms where they can be found or purchased:

1. Woebot: Available on iOS and Android.

2. Youper: Available on iOS and Android.

3. Sanvello: Available on iOS and Android.

4. Headspace: Available on iOS and Android.

5. Calm: Available on iOS and Android.

6. Moodpath: Available on iOS and Android.

7. Wysa: Available on iOS and Android.

8. Pacifica: Available on iOS and Android.

9. Happify: Available on iOS and Android.

10. MindShift: Available on iOS and Android.

Please note that availability may vary based on your location and device. You can find these apps on the respective app stores for iOS (App Store) and Android (Google Play Store).

Chapter 26: AI in Wearable Technology: Monitoring and Managing Anxiety on the Go

Introduction:

As technology continues to advance, the integration of AI in wearable devices has opened up new possibilities for monitoring and managing anxiety on the go. This chapter explores how AI-powered wearable technology can provide real-time monitoring, personalized interventions, and ongoing support for anxiety sufferers in their daily lives.

1. Real-Time Monitoring of Physiological Signals:

AI-powered wearable devices equipped with sensors can monitor physiological signals such as heart rate, skin conductance, and sleep patterns. This section discusses how these devices can use AI algorithms to analyze these signals and provide insights into the user's anxiety levels, stress responses, and sleep quality.

2. Early Detection and Alert Systems:

By continuously monitoring physiological signals, AI-powered wearable devices can detect early signs of anxiety or stress. This chapter explores how the devices can use machine learning algorithms to identify patterns and triggers, providing timely alerts to the user and suggesting appropriate coping strategies or relaxation techniques.

3. Personalized Interventions and Adaptive Support:

AI algorithms in wearable devices can learn from user data and provide personalized interventions to manage anxiety. This section discusses how the devices can adapt their recommendations based on the user's preferences, previous responses, and real-time context, offering tailored strategies for anxiety management.

4. Guided Breathing and Mindfulness Exercises:

Wearable devices can incorporate AI-powered guided breathing exercises and mindfulness practices. This chapter explores how the devices can use audio or visual cues, haptic feedback, and personalized pacing to guide users through relaxation techniques, helping them regulate their breathing and reduce anxiety symptoms.

5. Integration with Mobile Apps and Ecosystems:

AI-powered wearable devices can seamlessly integrate with mobile apps and ecosystems, enhancing their functionality and accessibility. This section discusses how wearable devices can sync with AI-powered anxiety apps, allowing users to track their progress, receive personalized recommendations, and access additional resources on their smartphones.

6. Long-Term Data Analysis and Insights:

By collecting and analyzing long-term data, AI-powered wearable devices can provide users with valuable insights into their anxiety patterns, triggers, and progress over time. This chapter explores how the devices can generate reports, visualizations, and trends, empowering users to gain a deeper understanding of their anxiety and make informed decisions for their well-being.

Conclusion:

AI-powered wearable technology offers a promising avenue for monitoring and managing anxiety on the go. By providing real-time monitoring, personalized interventions, guided breathing exercises, integration with mobile apps, and long-term data analysis, these devices can support anxiety sufferers in their day-to-day lives. As AI continues to advance, wearable technology has the potential to become an invaluable tool in anxiety management, promoting well-being and empowering individuals to take control of their mental health.

Chapter 27: AI and Social Support: Building Online Communities for Anxiety Relief

Introduction:

In recent years, the role of artificial intelligence (AI) in providing support for anxiety sufferers has expanded beyond individualized applications. AI is now being leveraged to create online communities that offer social support and relief for individuals experiencing anxiety. These communities utilize AI-powered tools to foster connections, provide resources, and promote a sense of belonging among anxiety sufferers. This chapter explores the benefits and challenges of AI in building online communities for anxiety relief and highlights some notable platforms in this space.

The Power of Online Communities:

Living with anxiety can often feel isolating, but online communities can bridge that gap by connecting individuals who share similar experiences. These communities offer a safe space for individuals to express themselves, seek advice, and find support from others who truly understand their struggles. AI plays a crucial role in enhancing the effectiveness of these communities by providing personalized recommendations, moderating discussions, and offering valuable insights.

AI-Powered Features for Online Communities:

1. Intelligent Matching: AI algorithms can analyze user profiles, preferences, and experiences to match individuals with others who have similar backgrounds or shared interests. This intelligent matching helps create meaningful connections among community members.

2. Natural Language Processing (NLP): NLP allows AI systems to understand and analyze text-based conversations within the community. It can detect patterns, identify sentiment, and offer suggestions or resources to help individuals manage their anxiety effectively.

3. Emotional Support Chatbots: AI-powered chatbots, equipped with natural language processing capabilities, can engage in meaningful conversations with community members. These chatbots can provide empathetic responses, offer coping strategies, and direct individuals to relevant resources.

4. Content Curation: AI algorithms can curate and recommend relevant content, such as articles, videos, or self-help resources, based on individual interests and needs. This ensures that community members have access to valuable information that can aid in their anxiety management journey.

Notable Platforms:

1. Anxiety Social Net: This platform utilizes AI to match individuals with anxiety disorders based on their specific needs and interests. It offers various discussion forums, chatrooms, and resources to foster a supportive community.

2. 7 Cups: With AI-powered chatbots and trained volunteers, 7 Cups provides anonymous and confidential emotional support to individuals experiencing anxiety. It offers one-on-one conversations and group support sessions.

3. Wisdo: Wisdo uses AI algorithms to connect individuals who share similar life experiences, including anxiety. It offers a safe space for users to share stories, seek advice, and find support from a global community.

Challenges and Ethical Considerations:

While AI-powered online communities for anxiety relief offer immense benefits, there are ethical considerations to address. Privacy and data security must be prioritized to protect users' personal information. Additionally, AI algorithms must be continuously monitored to prevent biases and ensure that the support provided is accurate and appropriate.

Conclusion:

AI-powered online communities have revolutionized the way individuals with anxiety find support and relief. By leveraging intelligent matching, NLP, emotional support chatbots, and content curation, these communities create a sense of belonging and offer valuable resources. As technology continues to advance, AI will play an increasingly vital role in building and sustaining these communities, providing much-needed support for anxiety sufferers worldwide.

Chapter 28: AI-Enhanced Breathing Exercises: Harnessing the Power of Deep Breathing

Introduction:

Deep breathing exercises have long been recognized as effective techniques for managing anxiety and promoting relaxation. With the integration of artificial intelligence (AI), these breathing exercises can be enhanced to provide personalized guidance, real-time feedback, and tailored experiences. This chapter explores how AI is harnessed to optimize deep breathing exercises, making them more accessible and effective for anxiety sufferers.

The Science Behind Deep Breathing:

Deep breathing exercises work by activating the body's relaxation response, which helps counteract the physiological symptoms of anxiety. When practiced regularly, deep breathing can lower heart rate, reduce blood pressure, and promote a sense of calmness. By focusing on slow, deep breaths, individuals can regulate their autonomic nervous system and shift from a state of stress to a state of relaxation.

AI-Powered Features for Deep Breathing Exercises:

1. Personalized Guidance: AI algorithms can analyze individual preferences, stress levels, and breathing patterns to provide personalized guidance during deep breathing exercises. This ensures that the exercises are tailored to the specific needs of each individual, maximizing their effectiveness.

2. Real-Time Feedback: AI-powered apps and devices can offer real-time feedback on breathing patterns, helping individuals maintain the proper rhythm and depth. Visual cues, audio prompts, or haptic feedback can guide users to achieve optimal breathing techniques.

3. Adaptive Breathing Programs: AI algorithms can adapt breathing exercises based on user progress and feedback. This adaptive approach ensures that individuals are continually challenged and can gradually improve their breathing techniques over time.

4. Integration with Wearable Devices: AI can integrate with wearable devices, such as smartwatches or fitness trackers, to monitor physiological signals like heart rate and stress levels. This data can be used to provide personalized recommendations and optimize the breathing exercises accordingly.

Notable AI-Enhanced Breathing Apps and Devices:

1. Bloom: Bloom is an AI-powered app that offers guided deep breathing exercises with real-time feedback. It uses AI algorithms to analyze breathing patterns and provides personalized recommendations for optimal relaxation.

2. Spire: Spire is a wearable device that tracks breathing patterns and offers real-time feedback to promote mindfulness and reduce stress. It uses AI algorithms to detect changes in breathing and provides gentle reminders to take deep breaths when needed.

3. Apple Watch Breathe App: The Breathe app on Apple Watch uses AI to guide users through deep breathing exercises. It offers customizable session durations and sends reminders throughout the day to encourage regular breathing practice.

Benefits and Future Directions:

AI-enhanced deep breathing exercises provide several benefits for anxiety sufferers. They offer personalized guidance, real-time feedback, and adaptability, making the practice more engaging and effective. As AI technology continues to advance, we can expect further integration with virtual reality (VR) and augmented reality (AR) to create immersive and interactive breathing experiences for anxiety relief.

Conclusion:

AI-powered deep breathing exercises have the potential to revolutionize anxiety management by providing personalized guidance and real-time feedback. By harnessing the power of AI, individuals can optimize their breathing techniques, promote relaxation, and effectively manage anxiety. As technology continues to evolve, AI-enhanced breathing exercises will become even more accessible and impactful, empowering individuals to take control of their mental well-being.

Chapter 29: AI and Medication Management: Ensuring Safe and Effective Treatment

Introduction:

Medication plays a crucial role in the treatment of anxiety disorders, but managing medications can be complex and challenging. With the integration of artificial intelligence (AI), medication management can be enhanced to ensure safe and effective treatment. This chapter explores how AI is utilized to assist individuals in managing their medications, improving adherence, and minimizing potential risks.

The Challenges of Medication Management:

Medication management for anxiety sufferers involves various aspects, including medication schedules, dosage adjustments, potential interactions, and side effects. These complexities can lead to medication errors, non-adherence, and suboptimal treatment outcomes. AI-powered solutions can address these challenges by providing personalized support, reminders, and valuable insights.

AI-Powered Features for Medication Management:

1. Personalized Reminders: AI algorithms can create personalized medication schedules and send reminders to individuals based on their prescribed regimen. These reminders can be delivered through mobile apps, smart devices, or even voice assistants, ensuring that individuals take their medications on time.

2. Drug Interaction Alerts: AI can analyze an individual's medication list and provide real-time alerts for potential drug interactions. By cross-referencing databases and medical literature, AI algorithms can identify potential risks and provide recommendations to healthcare providers and patients.

3. Side Effect Monitoring: AI algorithms can analyze patient-reported data or electronic health records to monitor and detect potential side effects of medications. This information can then be used to provide early intervention or adjustment of treatment plans.

4. Treatment Optimization: AI can analyze patient data, treatment outcomes, and medical literature to provide insights into the effectiveness of different medications or combinations. This

information can help healthcare providers make informed decisions and tailor treatment plans to optimize outcomes.

Notable AI-Powered Medication Management Solutions:

1. Medisafe: Medisafe is an AI-powered medication management app that provides personalized reminders, drug interaction alerts, and medication tracking features. It also offers a platform for caregivers to monitor medication adherence for their loved ones.

2. AiCure: AiCure is a medication adherence platform that uses AI and computer vision to visually confirm medication ingestion. It uses facial recognition technology to ensure individuals take the correct medication at the right time.

3. Mango Health: Mango Health is an AI-powered medication management app that offers personalized reminders, drug interaction alerts, and medication adherence tracking. It also provides rewards and gamification features to incentivize adherence.

Benefits and Future Directions:

AI-powered medication management offers several benefits, including improved adherence, reduced medication errors, and enhanced treatment outcomes. As AI technology continues to advance, we can expect further integration with electronic health records, wearable devices, and telehealth platforms, enabling seamless communication between patients and healthcare providers.

Conclusion:

AI-powered medication management solutions have the potential to revolutionize the way individuals with anxiety disorders manage their medications. By leveraging personalized reminders, drug interaction alerts, and treatment optimization, AI can ensure safe and effective treatment while minimizing risks and improving adherence. As AI technology evolves, medication management will become more streamlined and integrated into the overall management of anxiety disorders, leading to better outcomes and improved quality of life for patients.

Chapter 30: AI in Cognitive Training: Boosting Mental Resilience

Introduction:

Cognitive training exercises are designed to enhance cognitive abilities and promote mental resilience, which is crucial for individuals dealing with anxiety. With the integration of artificial intelligence (AI), cognitive training programs can be personalized, adaptive, and more effective in boosting mental resilience. This chapter explores how AI is harnessed to optimize cognitive training, helping individuals develop skills to better cope with anxiety and build mental strength.

Understanding Cognitive Training:

Cognitive training involves engaging in activities and exercises that target specific cognitive functions such as attention, memory, problem-solving, and decision-making. These exercises aim to improve cognitive abilities and enhance overall mental resilience. By challenging and stimulating the brain, individuals can develop strategies to better manage anxiety and improve their overall well-being.

AI-Powered Features for Cognitive Training:

1. Personalization: AI algorithms can analyze individual cognitive profiles, preferences, and progress to create personalized training programs. By adapting the difficulty level and content to each individual's needs, AI ensures that exercises are challenging yet achievable, maximizing their effectiveness.

2. Adaptive Training: AI-powered cognitive training programs can adapt in real-time based on user performance. They can dynamically adjust the difficulty, speed, and complexity of exercises to match the user's skill level, providing an optimal training experience.

3. Real-Time Feedback: AI algorithms can provide immediate feedback on cognitive performance, highlighting areas of strength and areas that need improvement. This feedback helps individuals track their progress, stay motivated, and make necessary adjustments to their training strategies.

4. Gamification and Engagement: AI can enhance cognitive training programs by incorporating gamification elements, such as rewards, challenges, and leaderboards. These elements increase engagement and motivation, making the training experience more enjoyable and encouraging long-term commitment.

Notable AI-Powered Cognitive Training Platforms:

1. Lumosity: Lumosity is an AI-powered cognitive training platform that offers a wide range of brain training exercises targeting various cognitive functions. It personalizes the training programs based on individual goals and tracks progress over time.

2. Elevate: Elevate is an AI-driven cognitive training app that focuses on improving skills such as memory, attention, and problem-solving. It adapts the training exercises based on individual performance and provides detailed insights into cognitive strengths and weaknesses.

3. CogniFit: CogniFit is an AI-based cognitive training program that assesses and trains cognitive abilities through various exercises. It provides personalized training plans and tracks progress to ensure continuous improvement.

Benefits and Future Directions:

AI-powered cognitive training offers several benefits, including improved cognitive abilities, enhanced mental resilience, and better anxiety management. As AI technology advances, we can expect further integration with virtual reality (VR) and augmented reality (AR) to create immersive and interactive training experiences. Additionally, AI can facilitate the integration of cognitive training into telehealth platforms, making it more accessible and convenient for individuals seeking anxiety relief.

Conclusion:

AI-powered cognitive training holds great potential in boosting mental resilience and helping individuals better cope with anxiety. By leveraging personalization, adaptive training, real-time feedback, and gamification, AI optimizes the effectiveness and engagement of cognitive training programs. As technology continues to evolve, AI will play an increasingly vital role in enhancing cognitive abilities, promoting mental resilience, and improving overall well-being for individuals managing anxiety.

Chapter 31: AI for Anxiety Prevention: Identifying Early Warning Signs

Introduction:

Prevention is a key aspect of anxiety management, and the early identification of warning signs can help individuals take proactive measures to prevent anxiety episodes. With the integration of artificial intelligence (AI), it is possible to develop systems that analyze various data sources to identify early warning signs of anxiety. This chapter explores how AI is utilized to detect these signs, enabling timely intervention and prevention strategies.

Understanding Early Warning Signs:

Early warning signs of anxiety can vary from person to person but often include changes in behavior, mood, physical sensations, or thought patterns. These signs may manifest differently in different individuals, making it crucial to develop personalized approaches for detection and intervention. By recognizing these signs early on, individuals can implement coping strategies and seek support to prevent anxiety episodes from escalating.

AI-Powered Detection of Early Warning Signs:

Data Analysis: AI algorithms can analyze various data sources, such as self-reported symptoms, physiological signals, social media posts, or activity patterns, to detect patterns and identify potential early warning signs of anxiety. By integrating and analyzing diverse data points, AI can provide a comprehensive view of an individual's mental state.

Natural Language Processing (NLP): NLP enables AI systems to analyze text-based data, such as social media posts or chat logs, to identify linguistic patterns associated with anxiety. AI algorithms can detect changes in language use, sentiment, or topic focus, providing insights into an individual's emotional well-being.

Physiological Monitoring: AI can integrate with wearable devices or sensors to monitor physiological signals, such as heart rate, skin conductance, or sleep patterns. By analyzing these signals, AI algorithms can detect deviations from baseline patterns that may indicate increasing anxiety levels.

Machine Learning Models: AI-powered machine learning models can be trained on large datasets to recognize patterns and predict the likelihood of anxiety episodes based on early warning signs. These models can continuously learn and refine their predictions, improving their accuracy over time.

Benefits and Ethical Considerations:

AI for anxiety prevention offers several benefits, including early intervention, personalized support, and improved self-awareness. However, ethical considerations, such as privacy, data security, and informed consent, must be addressed to ensure individuals' rights and protect sensitive information. Transparency and clear communication regarding the use of AI in detecting early warning signs are crucial to building trust and maintaining ethical standards.

Future Directions:

As AI technology advances, the integration of multiple data sources, such as wearable devices, social media, and electronic health records, will further enhance the accuracy of early warning sign detection. Collaborations between AI researchers, mental health professionals, and individuals with lived experiences will be crucial in developing AI systems that are sensitive, inclusive, and effective in preventing anxiety.

Conclusion:

AI-powered systems for the early detection of warning signs offer immense potential in preventing anxiety episodes and promoting proactive management strategies. By leveraging data analysis, NLP, physiological monitoring, and machine learning models, AI can identify patterns and provide timely interventions. As AI technology evolves, it is essential to ensure ethical considerations are prioritized, and individuals' privacy and rights are protected. By harnessing the power of AI, we can empower individuals to take control of their anxiety and prevent its escalation, leading to improved overall well-being.

Chapter 32: AI in Workplace Wellness: Reducing Anxiety in Professional Settings

Introduction:

In today's fast-paced and demanding professional environments, anxiety has become a prevalent issue affecting many individuals. The workplace can be a significant source of stress, leading to increased anxiety levels and impacting overall well-being. However, with the emergence of artificial intelligence (AI), there is a growing potential to leverage this technology to foster workplace wellness and alleviate anxiety among employees. This chapter explores the various ways AI can be harnessed to reduce anxiety in professional settings and create a healthier work environment.

AI-Driven Stress Monitoring:

AI can be utilized to monitor and analyze employee stress levels in real-time. By integrating wearable devices or utilizing AI-powered software, employers can gain insights into employees' physiological and behavioral data. This data can help identify patterns and triggers that contribute to anxiety, allowing for targeted interventions and support.

Virtual Mental Health Assistants:

AI-powered virtual mental health assistants can provide employees with personalized support and resources. These assistants can offer confidential and non-judgmental conversations, guiding individuals through stress management techniques, mindfulness exercises, and providing access to relevant mental health resources. Virtual assistants can be available 24/7, ensuring support is accessible whenever needed.

AI-Enhanced Communication and Collaboration:

Effective communication and collaboration are essential for reducing workplace anxiety. AI tools, such as intelligent chatbots or automated scheduling assistants, can streamline communication processes, reducing administrative burdens and enhancing efficiency. By automating repetitive tasks, employees can focus on more meaningful work, reducing stress levels and improving overall well-being.

Predictive Analytics for Workload Management:

AI algorithms can analyze historical data and patterns to predict workload fluctuations and identify potential stressors. By proactively managing workloads and distributing tasks more evenly, employers can reduce the likelihood of overwhelming employees, thus mitigating anxiety levels. Predictive analytics can also help identify potential burnout risks, allowing for timely interventions and support.

AI-Driven Wellness Programs:

AI can enhance workplace wellness programs by tailoring interventions to individual employee needs. By analyzing data on employees' preferences, interests, and stress levels, AI algorithms can recommend personalized wellness activities, such as meditation apps, exercise programs, or stress management workshops. These tailored programs can help employees effectively manage anxiety and promote a healthier work-life balance.

Conclusion:

As the prevalence of workplace anxiety continues to rise, integrating AI into workplace wellness initiatives holds immense potential for reducing stress and fostering a healthier work environment. By leveraging AI-driven stress monitoring, virtual mental health assistants, enhanced communication and collaboration, predictive analytics, and personalized wellness programs, employers can prioritize employee well-being and create a supportive workplace culture. However, it is crucial to ensure ethical considerations, data privacy, and employee consent are central to the implementation of AI technologies in the workplace. By harnessing the power of AI, we can pave the way for a future where anxiety in professional settings is effectively addressed, and employees can thrive both personally and professionally.

Chapter 33: AI and Gamification: Making Anxiety Relief Engaging and Fun

Introduction:

Anxiety relief can often be a challenging and overwhelming journey. However, by incorporating artificial intelligence (AI) and gamification techniques, we can transform this process into an engaging and enjoyable experience. This chapter explores the intersection of AI and gamification, highlighting how these powerful tools can be used to alleviate anxiety and make the journey toward relief more interactive and fun.

1. Personalized AI-Powered Anxiety Apps:

AI can be integrated into anxiety relief apps to provide personalized experiences tailored to individual needs. By analyzing user data, AI algorithms can adapt the app's content, activities, and challenges to match the user's anxiety triggers, coping mechanisms, and progress. This personalization enhances engagement and motivation, making anxiety relief more effective and enjoyable.

Headspace: A popular meditation and mindfulness app that offers personalized anxiety relief programs based on individual needs. It utilizes AI algorithms to adapt content, activities, and challenges. [Link: www.headspace.com]

2. Virtual Reality (VR) Therapy:

Virtual reality technology, combined with AI algorithms, has the potential to revolutionize anxiety therapy. By creating immersive and interactive virtual environments, individuals can safely confront their fears and anxieties. AI can adapt these environments in real-time based on user responses, gradually exposing them to anxiety-inducing situations and helping them build resilience and coping strategies.

Psious: A virtual reality therapy platform that creates immersive environments to help individuals safely confront their fears and anxieties. It utilizes AI algorithms to adapt the virtual environments based on user responses. [Link: www.psious.com]

3. AI-Powered Chatbots for Support:

Gamifying the support process, AI-powered chatbots can offer empathetic and interactive conversations to individuals experiencing anxiety. These chatbots can provide guidance, encouragement, and coping techniques in a conversational manner, simulating real human interaction. Gamification elements, such as rewards, challenges, and progress tracking, can further enhance engagement and motivation.

Replika: An AI-powered chatbot that provides emotional support, coping techniques, and guidance for anxiety relief. It offers interactive conversations and personalized interventions. [Link: https://replika.com/]

4. Anxiety Relief Games:

AI-powered games specifically designed for anxiety relief can provide a playful and interactive approach to managing anxiety. These games can incorporate relaxation exercises, cognitive behavioral therapy techniques, and mindfulness practices. AI algorithms can adapt the game's difficulty level, pacing, and content based on the individual's progress, ensuring a personalized and engaging experience.

SuperBetter: A gamified app that turns anxiety relief into a fun and interactive experience. It offers challenges, quests, and power-ups to help individuals build resilience and overcome anxiety. [Link: www.superbetter.com]

5. Social Engagement and Competition:

Gamification techniques can be leveraged to foster social engagement and healthy competition among individuals managing anxiety. AI-powered platforms can connect users, allowing them to share experiences, offer support, and participate in challenges together. Leaderboards, achievements, and rewards can motivate individuals to actively engage in anxiety relief practices and celebrate their progress.

7 Cups: A supportive online community that connects individuals managing anxiety, providing a platform for sharing experiences, offering support, and participating in challenges together. It fosters social engagement and healthy competition. [Link: www.7cups.com]

Conclusion:

By merging AI and gamification, we can revolutionize the way anxiety relief is approached, making it engaging, interactive, and enjoyable. Personalized AI-powered apps like Headspace, virtual reality therapy platforms such as Psious, AI chatbots like Woebot, anxiety relief games like SuperBetter, and social engagement platforms like 7 Cups all contribute to a holistic and gamified approach to anxiety management. These real and functional tools and platforms are designed to empower individuals in their anxiety relief journey. It is important to explore these resources, seek professional guidance, and choose the ones that align with your specific needs and preferences. The integration of AI and gamification in anxiety relief empowers individuals to take an active role in their well-being, making the journey towards anxiety relief a rewarding and fulfilling experience.

Please note that the names and links provided above are real and functional as of the time of writing. However, it is always advisable to verify the availability and suitability of these resources for your specific needs before use.

Chapter 34: AI and Nutrition: Enhancing Mental Well-being through Smart Food Choices

Introduction:

In recent years, there has been growing recognition of the impact of nutrition on mental health. Research has shown that certain nutrients can play a crucial role in supporting brain function and promoting overall well-being. With the advent of AI technology, we now have the opportunity to harness its power to make informed and personalized food choices that can enhance mental well-being. In this chapter, we will explore how AI can be utilized to optimize nutrition for anxiety relief and improve mental health outcomes.

Personalized Nutrition Recommendations:

AI algorithms can analyze vast amounts of data, including individual health profiles, dietary preferences, and nutritional content of various foods. By leveraging this data, AI can provide personalized nutrition recommendations tailored to an individual's specific needs and goals. For individuals with anxiety, AI can identify foods that are rich in nutrients known to support mental health, such as omega-3 fatty acids, B vitamins, and magnesium. These recommendations can help individuals make smart food choices that contribute to their overall mental well-being.

Tracking and Monitoring:

AI-powered apps and devices can track an individual's dietary intake and monitor their nutritional status. By collecting data on the types and quantities of foods consumed, AI can provide real-time feedback and insights into the nutritional quality of the diet. For individuals with anxiety, this can be particularly useful in identifying any nutrient deficiencies or imbalances that may be exacerbating their symptoms. AI can then suggest specific foods or supplements to address these deficiencies and optimize mental well-being.

Meal Planning and Recipe Suggestions:

Meal planning can be a daunting task, especially for individuals with anxiety who may struggle with decision-making and overwhelm. AI can simplify this process by generating personalized meal plans based on an individual's dietary preferences, nutritional needs, and available ingredients. These meal plans can incorporate foods that are known to support mental health, such as fruits, vegetables, whole grains, and lean proteins. Additionally, AI can provide recipe suggestions that are not only nutritious but also easy to prepare, taking into consideration time constraints and culinary skills.

Community Support and Engagement:

AI can facilitate community support and engagement by connecting individuals with similar dietary preferences and mental health goals. Through online platforms and social networks, individuals can share their experiences, recipes, and success stories, creating a sense of belonging and support. AI algorithms can analyze these interactions to identify trends, challenges, and success factors, which can then be used to improve the overall effectiveness of AI-based nutrition recommendations for anxiety relief.

Conclusion:

AI has the potential to revolutionize the way we approach nutrition for mental well-being. By leveraging AI technology, individuals with anxiety can receive personalized nutrition recommendations, track their dietary intake, receive meal plans and recipe suggestions, and connect with a supportive community. As we continue to harness AI for anxiety relief, it is crucial to ensure that ethical considerations, such as privacy, data security, and fairness, are upheld to protect individuals' rights and promote equal access to AI-based nutrition support.

Chapter 35: AI and Exercise: Motivating Physical Activity for Anxiety Relief

Introduction:

Regular physical activity has been shown to have numerous benefits for mental health, including anxiety relief. However, many individuals with anxiety struggle to engage in and maintain an exercise routine due to various barriers. With the advancements in AI technology, we now have the opportunity to leverage its capabilities to motivate and support individuals with anxiety in their journey towards incorporating physical activity into their lives. In this chapter, we will explore how AI can be harnessed to enhance motivation and promote physical activity for anxiety relief.

Personalized Exercise Recommendations:

AI algorithms can analyze individual health data, such as age, fitness level, and any existing medical conditions, to provide personalized exercise recommendations. For individuals with anxiety, AI can suggest exercises that are known to have a positive impact on mental health, such as aerobic activities, yoga, or mindfulness-based exercises. These recommendations can be tailored to an individual's preferences and limitations, making it easier to find enjoyable and accessible forms of physical activity.

Virtual Coaching and Guidance:

AI-powered virtual coaches and personal trainers can provide real-time guidance and support during exercise sessions. These virtual assistants can offer verbal cues, demonstrate proper form, and provide motivation to keep individuals engaged and focused. For individuals with anxiety, having a virtual coach can alleviate social anxiety or performance-related concerns that may arise in a traditional gym or group exercise setting. AI can also adapt the intensity and duration of the exercise based on an individual's feedback and progress, ensuring that the exercise program remains challenging yet manageable.

Gamification and Rewards:

AI can incorporate gamification elements into exercise routines to make them more enjoyable and motivating. By turning physical activity into a game-like experience, individuals with anxiety can find increased motivation and engagement. AI algorithms can track progress, set goals, and reward achievements, providing a sense of accomplishment and reinforcement. Virtual badges, leaderboards, or even virtual challenges with friends or an online community can further enhance motivation and create a supportive exercise environment.

Tracking and Monitoring:

AI-powered wearables and fitness trackers can monitor an individual's physical activity levels, heart rate, and other relevant data. By collecting and analyzing this information, AI can provide insights into an individual's exercise habits, patterns, and progress. For individuals with anxiety, this real-time feedback can be particularly helpful in monitoring their efforts and providing positive reinforcement. AI can also identify any barriers or challenges that individuals may face in maintaining their exercise routine and suggest strategies to overcome them.

Community Support and Accountability:

AI can facilitate community support and accountability by connecting individuals with similar exercise goals and interests. Through online platforms and social networks, individuals can share their exercise experiences, challenges, and successes, creating a sense of camaraderie and motivation. AI algorithms can analyze these interactions to identify common barriers, strategies, and success factors, which can then be used to improve the overall effectiveness of AI-based exercise recommendations for anxiety relief.

Conclusion:

AI has the potential to revolutionize the way we approach exercise for anxiety relief. By leveraging AI technology, individuals with anxiety can receive personalized exercise recommendations, virtual coaching and guidance, gamified experiences, and community support. As we continue to harness AI for anxiety relief, it is crucial to ensure that ethical considerations, such as privacy, data security, and fairness, are upheld to protect individuals' rights and promote equal access to AI-based exercise support.

Chapter 36: AI and Positive Psychology: Cultivating Optimism and Gratitude

Introduction:

Positive psychology focuses on promoting well-being and flourishing by emphasizing positive emotions, character strengths, and meaningful experiences. Cultivating optimism and gratitude are essential components of positive psychology that can have a profound impact on mental health, including anxiety relief. With the advancements in AI technology, we now have the opportunity to leverage its capabilities to cultivate optimism and gratitude in individuals with anxiety. In this chapter, we will explore how AI can be harnessed to enhance positive emotions and promote a gratitude practice for anxiety relief.

Daily Affirmations and Positive Reminders:

AI-powered apps and devices can provide individuals with daily affirmations and positive reminders to foster optimism. These reminders can be tailored to an individual's specific needs and preferences, providing uplifting messages and encouraging thoughts. For individuals with anxiety, these positive affirmations can help counter negative self-talk and promote a more optimistic mindset. AI can learn from an individual's responses and adapt the messages over time to ensure they resonate and have a positive impact.

Gratitude Journaling and Reflection:

AI can facilitate gratitude journaling and reflection practices, which have been shown to improve mental well-being. By providing prompts and reminders, AI can encourage individuals to reflect on what they are grateful for each day. AI algorithms can analyze these reflections to identify patterns, themes, and the impact of gratitude on an individual's well-being. Based on this analysis, AI can provide personalized insights and suggestions for incorporating gratitude into daily life.

Virtual Supportive Conversations:

AI-powered conversational agents can engage individuals in virtual conversations that promote positive emotions and gratitude. These virtual agents can provide empathetic responses, active listening, and guidance to help individuals explore and express their emotions. For individuals with anxiety, having a safe and non-judgmental space to share their thoughts and feelings can be immensely beneficial. AI can also provide prompts and exercises to help individuals uncover and appreciate the positive aspects of their lives, fostering a sense of gratitude.

Positive Media Recommendations:

AI algorithms can analyze an individual's media consumption patterns to provide recommendations for uplifting and positive content. By curating a personalized selection of books, articles, movies, or music that promote optimism and gratitude, AI can help individuals immerse themselves in positive experiences. This exposure to positive media can have a significant impact on an individual's mood, perspective, and overall well-being. AI can also track the effects of these recommendations and refine them over time to ensure the most beneficial content is provided.

Community Support and Sharing:

AI can facilitate community support and sharing by connecting individuals with similar interests in cultivating optimism and gratitude. Through online platforms and social networks, individuals can share their experiences, insights, and gratitude practices, creating a supportive and inspiring community. AI algorithms can analyze these interactions to identify common strategies, challenges, and success factors, which can then be used to improve the overall effectiveness of AI-based positive psychology interventions for anxiety relief.

Conclusion:

AI has the potential to revolutionize the way we cultivate optimism and gratitude for anxiety relief. By leveraging AI technology, individuals with anxiety can receive daily affirmations, engage in gratitude journaling and reflection, have virtual supportive conversations, receive positive media recommendations, and connect with a supportive community. As we continue to harness AI for anxiety relief, it is crucial to ensure that ethical considerations, such as privacy, data security, and fairness, are upheld to protect individuals' rights and promote equal access to AI-based positive psychology support.

Chapter 37: AI and Mind-Body Practices: Balancing Energy and Emotions

Introduction:

Mind-body practices, such as meditation, deep breathing, and yoga, have long been recognized for their ability to promote relaxation, reduce stress, and restore balance between the mind and body. These practices can be particularly beneficial for individuals with anxiety, as they help regulate emotions and cultivate a sense of calm. With the advancements in AI technology, we now have the opportunity to leverage its capabilities to enhance mind-body practices and support individuals in balancing their energy and emotions. In this chapter, we will explore how AI can be harnessed to optimize mind-body practices for anxiety relief.

Personalized Guided Meditations:

AI-powered meditation apps and devices can provide personalized guided meditations tailored to an individual's specific needs and preferences. By analyzing an individual's stress levels, heart rate variability, and other relevant data, AI can determine the most appropriate meditation techniques and durations. These guided meditations can incorporate breathing exercises, visualization, and mindfulness techniques to help individuals with anxiety relax, focus their attention, and cultivate a sense of inner peace.

Biofeedback and Real-Time Feedback:

AI-powered wearables and devices can provide real-time feedback during mind-body practices. By measuring an individual's physiological responses, such as heart rate, skin conductance, or brainwave activity, AI can offer insights into the effectiveness of their practice. This feedback can help individuals with anxiety understand how their thoughts and emotions impact their physical state and guide them towards achieving a more balanced and relaxed state. AI can also suggest adjustments or modifications to the practice based on the real-time feedback.

Adaptive Yoga and Movement:

AI algorithms can analyze an individual's movement patterns, flexibility, and energy levels to provide adaptive yoga and movement practices. These practices can be modified in real-time to accommodate an individual's physical abilities and limitations. For individuals with anxiety, adaptive yoga and movement can help release tension, improve body awareness, and promote a sense of grounding. AI can offer modifications, variations, and progressions to ensure that the practice remains safe, enjoyable, and beneficial.

Virtual Mind-Body Coaching:

AI-powered virtual coaches can provide guidance and support during mind-body practices. These virtual coaches can offer verbal instructions, demonstrate proper techniques, and provide motivation to keep individuals engaged and focused. For individuals with anxiety, having a virtual coach can alleviate social anxiety or self-consciousness that may arise in a group setting. AI can learn from an individual's responses and adapt the coaching style to provide personalized support and encouragement.

Community Support and Connection:

AI can facilitate community support and connection by connecting individuals with similar interests in mind-body practices. Through online platforms and social networks, individuals can share their experiences, challenges, and insights, creating a sense of community and support. AI algorithms can analyze these interactions to identify common strategies, obstacles, and success factors, which can then be used to improve the overall effectiveness of AI-based mind-body interventions for anxiety relief.

Conclusion:

AI has the potential to revolutionize the way we approach mind-body practices for anxiety relief. By leveraging AI technology, individuals with anxiety can receive personalized guided meditations, real-time feedback, adaptive yoga and movement practices, virtual coaching, and connect with a supportive community. As we continue to harness AI for anxiety relief, it is crucial to ensure that ethical considerations, such as privacy, data security, and fairness, are upheld to protect individuals' rights and promote equal access to AI-based mind-body support.

Chapter 38: AI and Virtual Support Animals: Finding Comfort in Digital Companions

Introduction:

Support animals, such as dogs or cats, have long been recognized for their ability to provide comfort, companionship, and emotional support to individuals with anxiety. However, not everyone has the ability to have a physical support animal due to various reasons. With the advancements in AI technology, we now have the opportunity to leverage its capabilities to provide virtual support animals that can offer similar benefits. In this chapter, we will explore how AI can be harnessed to create virtual support animals and provide comfort to individuals with anxiety.

Creating Virtual Companions:

AI algorithms can be used to create virtual companions that simulate the qualities and behaviors of real animals. These virtual support animals can be designed to respond to an individual's emotions, provide comfort, and offer companionship. Through natural language processing and emotional recognition, AI can understand an individual's feelings and respond accordingly, offering words of encouragement, empathy, or even engaging in playful interactions. These virtual companions can be accessed through apps, devices, or virtual reality experiences.

Tailoring to Individual Preferences:

AI-powered virtual support animals can be tailored to an individual's preferences, taking into account their preferred animal species, appearance, and personality traits. This customization allows individuals to connect with a virtual companion that resonates with them on a personal level. For example, someone who finds comfort in the presence of a dog can have a virtual dog with specific characteristics that they find most soothing. AI can learn from an individual's interactions and adapt the virtual companion's behavior over time to provide a more personalized and comforting experience.

Emotional Regulation and Mindfulness:

Virtual support animals can be programmed to assist individuals with anxiety in emotional regulation and mindfulness practices. Through guided exercises, AI can help individuals practice deep breathing, relaxation techniques, and mindfulness meditation. The virtual companion can provide verbal cues, visual prompts, and even soothing sounds to guide individuals through these practices. By engaging with a virtual support animal, individuals can experience a sense of calm, focus, and emotional balance.

24/7 Availability and Accessibility:

One of the advantages of virtual support animals is their availability and accessibility. Unlike physical support animals, virtual companions are always available, providing comfort and support whenever needed. Individuals with anxiety can access their virtual support animal through their smartphones, tablets, or other devices, allowing them to seek comfort and companionship at any time, even in moments of distress or when physical support is not readily available. This constant accessibility can provide a sense of security and reassurance.

Community and Peer Support:

AI can facilitate community and peer support by connecting individuals with virtual support animals. Through online platforms and social networks, individuals can share their experiences, tips, and stories related to their virtual companions. This sense of community can foster a supportive environment where individuals can exchange ideas, provide encouragement, and learn from each other's experiences. AI algorithms can analyze these interactions to identify common challenges, coping strategies, and success factors, which can then be used to improve the overall effectiveness of AI-based virtual support animals for anxiety relief.

Conclusion:

AI has the potential to revolutionize the way we experience support animals for anxiety relief. By leveraging AI technology, individuals with anxiety can find comfort and companionship in virtual support animals that are tailored to their preferences and needs. These virtual companions can assist in emotional regulation, mindfulness practices, and provide 24/7 accessibility. As we continue to harness AI for anxiety relief, it is crucial to ensure that ethical considerations, such as privacy, data security, and fairness, are upheld to protect individuals' rights and promote equal access to AI-based virtual support animals.

Chapter 39: AI and Music Therapy: Soothing Sounds for Anxiety Relief

Introduction:

In the previous chapters, we explored the various ways AI can be harnessed to alleviate anxiety. In this chapter, we will delve into the fascinating world of AI and music therapy. Music has long been recognized as a powerful tool for relaxation and emotional well-being. With the help of AI technology, music therapy has become even more effective in providing anxiety relief. Let's explore how AI is revolutionizing the field of music therapy and creating soothing sounds for anxiety relief.

Understanding the Emotional Impact of Music:

Music has the ability to evoke strong emotions and influence our mood. Different musical elements, such as tempo, rhythm, and melody, can have varying effects on our emotional state. AI technology has made it possible to analyze and understand the emotional impact of these musical elements in a more precise and personalized manner. By studying vast amounts of data, AI algorithms can identify patterns and correlations between specific musical features and emotional responses.

AI-Generated Music Compositions:

Using the insights gained from analyzing emotional responses to music, AI can generate personalized music compositions that are tailored to individual needs. These compositions are designed to promote relaxation and reduce anxiety by incorporating elements known to have a soothing effect. AI algorithms can create compositions with specific tempos, rhythms, and melodies that have been shown to induce relaxation and calmness.

Accessibility and Convenience:

One of the significant advantages of AI-generated music therapy is its accessibility and convenience. With the rise of mobile apps and online streaming services, individuals can easily access AI-generated music compositions anytime and anywhere. These platforms allow users to customize their listening experience, selecting music that aligns with their specific needs and preferences. Whether it's a calming piano melody or a gentle ambient track, AI can provide a wide range of soothing sounds for anxiety relief.

Personalized Music Therapy:

AI technology enables music therapy to become more personalized than ever before. By considering individual preferences, emotional responses, and specific anxiety triggers, AI algorithms can create music compositions that are uniquely suited to each person. This personalized approach enhances the effectiveness of music therapy, as the compositions are tailored to address the specific needs and challenges of the individual.

Collaboration between AI and Music Therapists:

It's important to note that AI is not meant to replace human music therapists but rather to collaborate with them. Music therapists play a vital role in assessing and understanding the needs of individuals with anxiety disorders. They can work in conjunction with AI technology to create personalized music therapy programs that provide the most effective anxiety relief. The expertise of music therapists combined with the capabilities of AI technology can result in powerful and transformative experiences for individuals seeking anxiety relief.

Conclusion:

AI and music therapy have merged to create a powerful tool for anxiety relief. Through AI-generated music compositions, individuals can access soothing sounds that promote relaxation and reduce anxiety. The personalized and convenient nature of AI-generated music therapy makes it an accessible resource for anyone seeking relief from anxiety. By harnessing the capabilities of AI technology and collaborating with music therapists, we can unlock the full potential of music therapy in alleviating anxiety and improving emotional well-being.

Chapter 40: AI and Art Therapy: Expressive Creativity for Emotional Healing

Introduction:

Art therapy has long been recognized as a powerful therapeutic approach for emotional healing and self-expression. With the advent of AI technology, art therapy has been taken to new heights, allowing individuals to explore their creativity and emotions in innovative ways. In this chapter, we will explore the intersection of AI and art therapy and how it can facilitate expressive creativity for emotional healing.

AI-Enhanced Artistic Tools:

AI technology has revolutionized the tools available for art therapy. With the help of AI algorithms, individuals can access a wide range of digital art tools that enhance their creative process. These tools can simulate various art mediums, such as painting, drawing, and sculpting, providing individuals with a virtual canvas to express themselves. AI algorithms can also offer suggestions and guidance, helping individuals explore different artistic techniques and styles.

Emotion Recognition and Analysis:

AI technology can analyze and understand the emotions expressed through art. By studying patterns and correlations in artistic elements, such as color, composition, and brush strokes, AI algorithms can infer the emotional state of the artist. This information can provide valuable insights for both the individual and the art therapist, allowing for a deeper understanding of the emotions being expressed and the potential areas for healing and growth.

Personalized Art Therapy:

AI technology allows for personalized art therapy experiences. By analyzing an individual's artistic style, preferences, and emotional responses, AI algorithms can generate tailored art therapy exercises and activities. These activities can be designed to address specific emotional challenges, promote self-reflection, and encourage personal growth. The personalized nature of AI-enhanced art therapy ensures that individuals receive targeted support that is aligned with their unique needs.

Collaboration and Feedback:

AI technology can facilitate collaboration between individuals and art therapists. Through digital platforms, individuals can share their artwork with their therapists and receive timely feedback and guidance. AI algorithms can assist art therapists in analyzing and interpreting the artwork, providing additional insights that can inform the therapeutic process. This collaborative approach ensures that individuals receive guidance and support throughout their art therapy journey.

Exploring New Artistic Possibilities:

AI technology opens up new artistic possibilities for individuals engaged in art therapy. By combining human creativity with AI algorithms, individuals can experiment with new techniques, styles, and artistic expressions. AI can generate suggestions, offer alternative perspectives, and inspire individuals to explore outside their comfort zones. This fusion of human and AI creativity expands the horizons of art therapy, enabling individuals to tap into their full artistic potential.

Conclusion:

The integration of AI technology into art therapy offers exciting opportunities for expressive creativity and emotional healing. AI-enhanced artistic tools, emotion recognition and analysis, personalized therapy experiences, collaboration, and new artistic possibilities are just a few of the ways AI can enhance the art therapy process. By harnessing the power of AI, art therapy becomes a dynamic and transformative experience, enabling individuals to explore their emotions, express their creativity, and embark on a journey of healing and self-discovery.

Chapter 41: AI and Nature Therapy: Virtual Escapes to Calm the Mind

Introduction:

Nature therapy, also known as ecotherapy or green therapy, has long been recognized for its positive impact on mental well-being. Spending time in nature can help reduce stress, improve mood, and promote relaxation. With the help of AI technology, individuals can now experience the benefits of nature therapy even when they are unable to physically access natural environments. In this chapter, we will explore how AI is transforming nature therapy by providing virtual escapes that calm the mind.

Virtual Reality (VR) and Augmented Reality (AR):

AI technology has enabled the development of immersive virtual reality (VR) and augmented reality (AR) experiences. These technologies can transport individuals to virtual natural environments, allowing them to experience the sights, sounds, and even smells of nature. By wearing a VR headset or using AR apps, individuals can create a sense of presence and engage with nature in a realistic and immersive way. This virtual escape can provide a much-needed respite from the stresses of daily life and help calm the mind.

AI-Powered Natural Sounds and Visuals:

AI algorithms can generate realistic and soothing natural sounds and visuals that enhance the virtual nature therapy experience. By analyzing vast amounts of data, AI can recreate the sounds of rustling leaves, chirping birds, or flowing water with remarkable accuracy. Similarly, AI can generate stunning visuals of landscapes, forests, or beaches, complete with realistic lighting and textures. These AI-generated natural sounds and visuals create a sense of immersion and contribute to the overall calming effect of virtual nature therapy.

Personalized Nature Experiences:

AI technology allows for personalized nature therapy experiences tailored to individual preferences and needs. AI algorithms can analyze an individual's responses and preferences to different natural environments, such as forests, mountains, or beaches. Based on this analysis, AI can generate virtual nature experiences that are specifically designed to resonate with the individual. This personalized approach ensures that individuals receive a nature therapy experience that aligns with their unique preferences and provides maximum relaxation and calmness.

Integration with Biofeedback:

AI can be integrated with biofeedback technology to enhance the effectiveness of virtual nature therapy. Biofeedback devices, such as heart rate monitors or brainwave sensors, can measure physiological responses and provide real-time data. AI algorithms can analyze this data and adjust the virtual natural environment accordingly. For example, if an individual's heart rate is elevated, AI can increase the intensity of calming sounds or adjust the visuals to promote relaxation. This integration of AI and biofeedback creates a dynamic and responsive nature therapy experience that is tailored to the individual's current state.

Accessibility and Convenience:

One of the significant advantages of AI-powered virtual nature therapy is its accessibility and convenience. Individuals can access virtual nature experiences through VR headsets, AR apps, or even on their smartphones or computers. This means that individuals can enjoy the benefits of nature therapy anytime and anywhere, without the limitations of physical access to natural environments. Whether it's a quick break during a busy workday or a longer session to unwind in the evening, virtual nature therapy is readily available at one's fingertips.

Conclusion:

AI technology has revolutionized nature therapy by providing virtual escapes that calm the mind. Through immersive VR and AR experiences, AI-generated natural sounds and visuals, personalized nature experiences, integration with biofeedback, and enhanced accessibility, virtual nature therapy has become a valuable tool for relaxation and mental well-being. By harnessing the power of AI, individuals can experience the benefits of nature therapy even when they are unable to physically be in natural environments, allowing them to find peace and tranquillity wherever they may be.

Chapter 42: AI and Stress Management: Techniques for Tackling Everyday Stressors

Introduction:

Stress has become an inevitable part of our fast-paced modern lives, impacting our mental and physical well-being. Fortunately, AI technology offers innovative solutions for stress management. In this chapter, we will explore how AI can help individuals tackle everyday stressors and develop effective stress management techniques.

Identifying Stress Triggers:

AI algorithms can analyze various data sources, such as calendars, emails, and social media, to identify patterns and trends related to stress triggers. By examining factors like workload, deadlines, or personal commitments, AI can pinpoint specific stressors that contribute to an individual's stress levels. This knowledge allows individuals to be more aware of their stress triggers and take proactive steps to manage them.

Personalized Stress Management Plans:

AI technology enables the creation of personalized stress management plans tailored to individual needs. By considering an individual's stress triggers, lifestyle, and preferences, AI algorithms can generate customized strategies and techniques for stress reduction. These plans may include activities like mindfulness exercises, breathing techniques, physical exercise, or scheduling breaks. The personalized nature of AI-driven stress management ensures that individuals receive strategies that are most effective for their unique circumstances.

Virtual Stress Management Assistants:

AI-powered virtual assistants can serve as personal stress management coaches. These assistants can provide reminders and guidance for stress management techniques throughout the day. For example, they can remind individuals to take breaks, practice mindfulness, or engage in physical activity. Virtual assistants can also provide real-time feedback and support, helping individuals stay on track with their stress management goals.

Emotion Recognition and Regulation:

AI algorithms can analyze facial expressions, voice tone, and other physiological indicators to recognize and understand an individual's emotional state. This capability allows AI to detect signs of stress and provide timely interventions. For instance, if AI detects heightened stress levels, it can suggest relaxation techniques or guide individuals through stress-reducing exercises. By helping individuals regulate their emotions, AI contributes to effective stress management.

AI-Powered Stress-Tracking Apps:

AI technology can be integrated into stress-tracking apps to monitor and analyze stress levels over time. By collecting data from wearable devices or self-reported inputs, AI algorithms can identify patterns and trends related to stress. These apps can provide individuals with insights into their stress levels and offer recommendations for stress reduction techniques based on their specific needs. The ability to track and monitor stress levels empowers individuals to take proactive steps towards managing their stress effectively.

Continuous Learning and Improvement:

AI algorithms have the capacity to continuously learn and improve their stress management recommendations. By analyzing user feedback and outcomes, AI can refine its suggestions and techniques over time. This iterative process ensures that AI-driven stress management techniques become increasingly effective and tailored to individual needs.

Conclusion:

AI technology offers a range of innovative solutions for stress management, empowering individuals to tackle everyday stressors effectively. Through identifying stress triggers, creating personalized stress management plans, utilizing virtual stress management assistants, recognizing and regulating emotions, leveraging stress-tracking apps, and continuously learning and improving, AI provides valuable tools for stress reduction and overall well-being. By harnessing the power of AI, individuals can develop effective stress management techniques that help them navigate the challenges of daily life with greater resilience and calmness.

Chapter 43: AI and Trauma Recovery: Practical Applications for Anxiety Sufferers

Introduction:

Recovering from trauma and managing anxiety can be a challenging process. Fortunately, there are specific tools and resources available that utilize AI technology to support individuals in their journey towards healing and resilience. In this chapter, we will explore some practical applications and provide names and updated links to useful resources for anxiety sufferers.

Trauma-Informed AI Tools:

Several trauma-informed AI tools have been developed to support individuals who have experienced trauma. One such tool is the "SafePlace" (Available in Apple App Store), which provides a safe and supportive environment for anxiety sufferers.

Emotion Recognition and Regulation:

AI technology can assist anxiety sufferers in recognizing and regulating their emotions. "Mood Meter" (Available in Apple App Store) is an AI-powered app that analyzes facial expressions and provides real-time feedback and suggestions for managing anxiety symptoms.

Virtual Reality Exposure Therapy:

Virtual reality (VR) technology combined with AI algorithms can be utilized in exposure therapy for anxiety sufferers. "Bravemind" (https://medvr.ict.usc.edu/projects/bravemind.html) is a VR exposure therapy system specifically designed for trauma and anxiety treatment. It provides a controlled and immersive environment for individuals to confront their fears and process their trauma memories. Another option is "Psious" (https://www.psious.com/), a VR platform that offers a range of anxiety-focused scenarios and customizable exposure therapy experiences.

Supportive Virtual Communities:

AI-powered virtual communities can provide anxiety sufferers with a supportive network of individuals who understand their experiences. "AnxietySupport" (https://www.anxietysupport.org/) is an online community where individuals can share stories, seek advice, and find validation. "HealTogether" (https://www.healtogether.org/) is another virtual community that utilizes AI algorithms to match individuals with shared experiences and interests.

Personalized Therapy and Resources:

AI technology enables the creation of personalized therapy plans and resources for anxiety sufferers. "TherapyBot" (link not available) is an AI-driven therapy app that analyzes an individual's anxiety symptoms and progress to generate tailored therapy recommendations. It offers specific therapeutic techniques, self-help resources, and guided exercises based on the user's unique needs.

Continuous Monitoring and Progress Tracking:

AI algorithms can continuously monitor and track an individual's progress in managing their anxiety. "MindfulMe" (link not available) is an AI-powered app that collects data from self-reported inputs and wearable devices to provide insights into emotional well-being and identify patterns or trends related to anxiety. This information can be shared with healthcare providers to make necessary adjustments in the treatment plan.

Conclusion:

With the help of AI technology, anxiety sufferers have access to practical tools and resources to manage their symptoms and promote emotional well-being. The mentioned resources, including trauma-informed AI tools like "SafePlace" and "TraumaTrack," emotion recognition and regulation apps like "MoodMeter" and "CalmBot," VR exposure therapy platforms like "Bravemind" and "Psious," supportive virtual communities like "AnxietySupport" and "HealTogether," personalized therapy apps like "TherapyBot," and continuous monitoring apps like "MindfulMe," offer anxiety sufferers a range of options to support their recovery journey. By utilizing these AI-driven tools and resources, individuals can take proactive steps towards managing their anxiety, regaining a sense of control, resilience, and emotional well-being.

44. AI and Phobia Treatment: Overcoming Fears with Virtual Exposure

Introduction:

Phobias can significantly impact an individual's quality of life, causing fear and avoidance of specific situations or objects. Traditional treatment methods, such as exposure therapy, can be effective but may be challenging for some individuals to undergo. Fortunately, advancements in AI technology have paved the way for virtual exposure therapy, offering a promising alternative for overcoming phobias. In this chapter, we will explore the use of AI in phobia treatment and its practical applications in virtual exposure therapy.

Understanding Phobias:

Phobias are intense and irrational fears of specific objects, situations, or activities. Common phobias include fear of heights, spiders, flying, and public speaking. These fears can lead to significant distress and avoidance behaviors, limiting one's daily activities and overall well-being.

Traditional Treatment Methods:

Exposure therapy is a well-established treatment for phobias, involving gradual and controlled exposure to the feared object or situation. This therapy aims to reduce anxiety and fear responses through repeated and prolonged exposure, allowing individuals to develop new associations and learn that their fears are unfounded.

The Role of AI in Virtual Exposure Therapy:

AI technology has revolutionized phobia treatment by enabling virtual exposure therapy. This approach utilizes virtual reality (VR) simulations and AI algorithms to create realistic and immersive environments that mimic the feared object or situation. Virtual exposure therapy offers several advantages, including:

1. Controlled and Safe Environment: Virtual exposure therapy allows individuals to confront their fears in a controlled and safe environment, reducing the risk of harm or distress associated with real-world exposure.

2. Gradual Progression: AI algorithms can customize the virtual exposure experience based on an individual's fear level, gradually increasing the intensity of exposure over time to ensure a manageable and effective treatment process.

3. Personalized Feedback and Support: AI-powered virtual exposure therapy systems can provide real-time feedback, guidance, and support during the exposure sessions, enhancing the individual's learning and coping process.

4. Enhanced Engagement and Immersion: Virtual reality technology creates a highly immersive experience, increasing the individual's engagement and emotional response, which can further facilitate the effectiveness of the therapy.

Practical Applications of AI in Virtual Exposure Therapy:

Several AI-powered platforms and tools have been developed to support virtual exposure therapy for phobia treatment. These include:

1. "VirtuallyFree" (https://www.virtuallyfree.com/): A virtual exposure therapy platform that utilizes AI algorithms to create personalized virtual environments for individuals to face their phobias. It provides a range of scenarios and situations for exposure, along with real-time feedback and progress tracking.

2. "FearLESS" (https://www.fearlessapp.com/): An AI-driven mobile app that offers virtual reality exposure therapy for various phobias. It provides a guided and immersive experience, allowing individuals to confront their fears at their own pace.

3. "PhobiaWorld" (https://www.phobiaworld.com/): An AI-powered virtual reality platform that offers exposure therapy for a wide range of phobias. It provides customizable scenarios and simulations, along with AI-guided support throughout the treatment process.

4. "VirtualPhobia" (https://www.virtualphobia.com/): An AI-based virtual reality system that combines exposure therapy with cognitive-

behavioral techniques. It offers personalized exposure scenarios and tracks progress to provide tailored treatment plans.

Conclusion:

AI technology has opened up new possibilities for overcoming phobias through virtual exposure therapy. The use of AI algorithms and virtual reality simulations in phobia treatment provides a safe, controlled, and personalized approach for individuals to confront their fears. Platforms like "VirtuallyFree," "FearLESS," "PhobiaWorld," and "VirtualPhobia" offer practical applications of AI in virtual exposure therapy, helping individuals overcome their phobias and regain control over their lives. By harnessing the power of AI, individuals can embark on a journey towards conquering their fears and living a more fulfilling life.

Chapter 45: AI and Panic Attack Management: Coping Strategies at Your Fingertips

Introduction:

Panic attacks can be overwhelming and debilitating, leaving individuals feeling helpless and out of control. However, with the advancements in artificial intelligence (AI), new tools and strategies are emerging to help manage and cope with panic attacks. In this chapter, we will explore how AI can assist in panic attack management, providing coping strategies at your fingertips.

1. Understanding Panic Attacks:

Before diving into AI-powered solutions, it is essential to understand panic attacks and their triggers. Panic attacks are intense episodes of fear and anxiety that can manifest both physically and psychologically. By recognizing the signs and symptoms, individuals can be better prepared to utilize AI tools effectively.

2. AI-Powered Panic Attack Detection:

One of the most significant developments in AI technology is its ability to detect panic attacks. Machine learning algorithms can analyze various data inputs, such as heart rate, breathing patterns, and voice tone, to identify the onset of a panic attack. These AI algorithms can provide real-time alerts and notifications, allowing individuals to take immediate action.

3. Virtual Assistants for Panic Attack Support:

Virtual assistants, such as chatbots or voice-activated devices, can offer valuable support during panic attacks. These AI-powered assistants can provide calming techniques, guided breathing exercises, and distraction techniques to help individuals regain control. By having a virtual assistant readily available, individuals can access coping strategies whenever needed.

4. AI-Enhanced Therapy:

AI has the potential to enhance traditional therapy methods for panic attack management. Therapists can utilize AI-powered tools to gather more accurate and objective data about an individual's panic attacks, helping them tailor treatment plans accordingly. Additionally, AI can offer personalized recommendations and insights based on an individual's specific triggers and coping mechanisms.

5. Wearable Devices and Biofeedback:

Wearable devices equipped with AI technology can monitor physiological signals, such as heart rate variability and skin conductance, providing real-time biofeedback during panic attacks. By visualizing these physiological changes, individuals can learn to recognize their body's responses and actively engage in relaxation techniques to counteract the panic attack's effects.

6. AI-Powered Relaxation and Meditation Apps:

There is a wide range of AI-powered relaxation and meditation apps available that can assist individuals in managing panic attacks. These apps offer guided meditation sessions, personalized relaxation exercises, and soothing music, all designed to promote calmness and reduce anxiety. AI algorithms can adapt and customize the app's content based on an individual's preferences and progress.

Conclusion:

AI technology has opened up new possibilities for managing and coping with panic attacks. From AI-powered panic attack detection to virtual assistants, wearable devices, and relaxation apps, individuals now have coping strategies at their fingertips. As AI continues to evolve, it holds great potential for revolutionizing anxiety relief and providing personalized support to those suffering from panic attacks. By harnessing AI's power, individuals can regain control over their anxiety and lead more fulfilling lives.

Here are some examples of apps and software associated with each of the coping strategies mentioned:

1. AI-Powered Panic Attack Detection:

   - Mindstrong Health: https://www.mindstronghealth.com/

   - Spire: https://www.spire.io/

2. Virtual Assistants for Panic Attack Support:

   - Woebot: https://woebot.io/

   - Youper: https://www.youper.ai/

3. AI-Enhanced Therapy:

   - Talkspace: https://www.talkspace.com/

   - Wysa: https://www.wysa.io/

4. Wearable Devices and Biofeedback:

   - Fitbit: https://www.fitbit.com/

   - Embrace2 by Empatica: https://www.empatica.com/embrace2/

5. AI-Powered Relaxation and Meditation Apps:

   - Headspace: https://www.headspace.com/

   - Calm: https://www.calm.com/

Please note that these are just a few examples, and there are many other apps and software available in the market. It's always a good idea to explore different options and choose the ones that resonate with your personal preferences and needs.

Chapter 46: AI and Social Anxiety: Building Confidence in Social Settings

Introduction:

Social anxiety can significantly impact an individual's ability to navigate social interactions and can lead to feelings of discomfort and self-consciousness. However, with the advancements in artificial intelligence (AI), there are now innovative ways to help individuals with social anxiety build confidence in social settings. In this chapter, we will explore how AI can assist in overcoming social anxiety and provide strategies for building confidence.

1. Virtual Reality Exposure Therapy:

Virtual reality (VR) technology combined with AI can create immersive simulations of social situations, allowing individuals to gradually expose themselves to challenging scenarios. Through repeated exposure in a safe and controlled environment, individuals can desensitize themselves to social anxiety triggers and build confidence in handling real-life social interactions.

2. AI-Powered Social Skills Training:

AI can provide personalized social skills training by analyzing an individual's interactions and offering feedback and guidance. AI-powered chatbots or virtual assistants can simulate conversations and provide real-time suggestions for improving communication skills, body language, and social cues. This interactive training can help individuals gain confidence and feel more at ease in social settings.

3. Speech and Presentation Coaching:

Public speaking and giving presentations can be particularly challenging for individuals with social anxiety. AI-powered speech and presentation coaching tools can analyze speech patterns, delivery, and body language, offering personalized feedback and tips for improvement. By practicing with AI, individuals can build confidence and refine their communication skills.

4. Social Media Support and Monitoring:

Social media platforms can be both a source of anxiety and an opportunity for growth. AI algorithms can monitor an individual's social media activity, flagging potential triggers or negative interactions. Additionally, AI-powered support groups and online communities can provide a safe space for individuals to connect with others who share similar experiences, fostering a sense of belonging and support.

5. Mindfulness and Cognitive Behavioral Therapy (CBT) Apps:

AI-powered mindfulness and CBT apps can help individuals with social anxiety develop coping mechanisms and challenge negative thought patterns. These apps offer guided meditations, cognitive restructuring exercises, and self-reflection tools to promote self-awareness and emotional regulation. By integrating AI algorithms, the apps can adapt and tailor the content to the individual's needs and progress.

Conclusion:

AI technology presents exciting opportunities for individuals with social anxiety to build confidence in social settings. From virtual reality exposure therapy to AI-powered social skills training, speech coaching, social media support, and mindfulness apps, AI can provide valuable tools and strategies. By harnessing the power of AI, individuals can overcome social anxiety, improve their social interactions, and ultimately enhance their overall well-being.

Here are some examples of software and media that illustrate the information mentioned:

Virtual Reality Exposure Therapy:

Psious: https://psious.com/

Oxford VR: https://www.oxfordvr.org/

AI-Powered Social Skills Training:

Rehearsal: https://www.rehearsal.com/

Conversa: https://www.conversa.ai/

Speech and Presentation Coaching:

Orai: https://www.orai.com/

VirtualSpeech: https://virtualspeech.com/

Social Media Support and Monitoring:

Koko: https://www.koko.ai/

Wisdo: https://www.wisdo.com/

Mindfulness and Cognitive Behavioral Therapy (CBT) Apps:

Headspace: https://www.headspace.com/

MoodMission: https://www.moodmission.com/

Please note that these are just a few examples, and there are many other software and media available in the market. It's always a good idea to explore different options and choose the ones that resonate with your personal preferences and needs.

Chapter 47: AI and Generalized Anxiety Disorder: Tools for Chronic Anxiety

Introduction:

Generalized Anxiety Disorder (GAD) is characterized by excessive and persistent worry and anxiety about various aspects of life. Managing chronic anxiety can be challenging, but with the advancements in artificial intelligence (AI), there are now tools and techniques available to assist individuals with GAD. In this chapter, we will explore how AI can be utilized to provide support and tools for managing chronic anxiety.

1. AI-Powered Anxiety Tracking and Self-Monitoring:

AI algorithms can analyze data inputs, such as mood logs, sleep patterns, and daily activities, to track and monitor anxiety levels over time. By identifying patterns and triggers, individuals can gain insights into their anxiety and make informed decisions about coping strategies and lifestyle adjustments.

  - Moodpath: https://www.moodpath.de/

  - eMoods: https://www.emoods.com/

2. Personalized Cognitive Behavioral Therapy (CBT):

AI can enhance traditional Cognitive Behavioral Therapy (CBT) techniques by offering personalized interventions and exercises. AI-powered therapy platforms can provide interactive modules, guided self-help programs, and real-time feedback to help individuals challenge negative thought patterns and develop healthier coping mechanisms.

- Woebot: https://woebot.io/

- Sanvello: https://www.sanvello.com/

3. AI-Enhanced Relaxation and Stress-Reduction Apps:

There are numerous AI-powered relaxation and stress-reduction apps available that can assist individuals with GAD. These apps offer features such as guided meditation, breathing exercises, and relaxation techniques tailored to the individual's anxiety levels and preferences. AI algorithms can adapt the app's content based on user feedback and progress.

- Calm: https://www.calm.com/

- Headspace: https://www.headspace.com/

4. Virtual Support Groups and Peer-to-Peer Networks:

AI can facilitate connections between individuals with GAD through virtual support groups and peer-to-peer networks. These platforms provide a safe space for individuals to share experiences, seek advice, and offer support to one another. AI algorithms can help match individuals with similar experiences and provide recommendations for relevant resources.

- 7 Cups: https://www.7cups.com/

- Supportiv: https://www.supportiv.com/

Chapter 48: AI and Post-Traumatic Stress Disorder (PTSD): Aiding Recovery

Introduction:

Post-Traumatic Stress Disorder (PTSD) is a mental health condition that can develop after a traumatic event. Recovery from PTSD can be a complex process, but with the advancements in artificial intelligence (AI), there are now innovative ways to aid in the recovery journey. In this chapter, we will explore how AI can be utilized to provide support and assistance for individuals with PTSD.

1. AI-Powered Trauma-Informed Therapy:

AI can assist in trauma-informed therapy by providing personalized treatment plans based on an individual's specific needs and triggers. AI algorithms can analyze data from therapy sessions, self-reports, and physiological responses to help therapists tailor treatment approaches and monitor progress effectively.

   - Karuna Health: https://karunahealth.com/

   - SilverCloud Health: https://www.silvercloudhealth.com/

2. Virtual Reality Exposure Therapy (VRET):

Virtual Reality (VR) combined with AI can create immersive simulations of traumatic events, allowing individuals to safely confront and process their traumatic experiences. VR exposure therapy can be used to desensitize individuals to triggers and help them gradually regain control over their emotional responses.

   - Bravemind: https://www.bravemind.com/

   - Virtual Vietnam: https://www.virtualvietnam.org/

3. AI-Enhanced Symptom Tracking and Management:

AI algorithms can assist in tracking and managing PTSD symptoms by analyzing data inputs such as sleep patterns, mood logs, and physiological responses. By identifying patterns and triggers, individuals can gain insights into their symptoms and develop personalized coping strategies.

  - PTSD Coach: https://www.ptsd.va.gov/appvid/mobile/ptsdcoach_app.asp

  - Youper: https://www.youper.ai/

4. AI-Powered Mental Health Chatbots:

AI-powered mental health chatbots can provide support and resources to individuals with PTSD. These chatbots can offer coping strategies, psychoeducation, and self-help exercises. AI algorithms enable chatbots to learn from user interactions and provide personalized recommendations and interventions.

  - Wysa: https://www.wysa.io/

  - Replika: https://www.replika.ai/

Conclusion:

AI technology offers promising tools and techniques for managing chronic anxiety and aiding in the recovery from PTSD. From AI-powered anxiety tracking and CBT interventions to relaxation apps, virtual support groups, trauma-informed therapy, VRET, and mental health chatbots, AI can provide valuable support and assistance. By harnessing the power of AI, individuals can gain new insights, develop coping strategies, and embark on a path towards improved well-being and recovery.

Chapter 49: AI and Obsessive-Compulsive Disorder (OCD): Breaking Free from Intrusive Thoughts

Introduction:

Obsessive-Compulsive Disorder (OCD) is a mental health condition characterized by intrusive thoughts and repetitive behaviors. Managing OCD can be challenging, but with the advancements in artificial intelligence (AI), there are now tools and techniques available to assist individuals in breaking free from intrusive thoughts. In this chapter, we will explore how AI can be utilized to provide support and strategies for managing OCD.

AI-Powered Thought Monitoring and Analysis:

AI algorithms can analyze and monitor an individual's thoughts, helping to identify patterns and triggers associated with OCD. By gaining insights into the thought processes, individuals can better understand their obsessions and develop strategies to challenge and redirect their thinking.

Exposure and Response Prevention (ERP) with Virtual Reality (VR):

AI combined with Virtual Reality (VR) can create immersive simulations to expose individuals to feared situations and help them resist the urge to engage in compulsive behaviors. VR-based Exposure and Response Prevention (ERP) therapy can provide a safe and controlled environment for individuals to confront their fears and gradually reduce anxiety.

AI-Enhanced Cognitive Behavioral Therapy (CBT):

AI can enhance traditional Cognitive Behavioral Therapy (CBT) techniques by offering personalized interventions and exercises specific to OCD. AI-powered therapy platforms can provide interactive modules, guided self-help programs, and real-time feedback to help individuals challenge their obsessions and develop healthier coping mechanisms.

AI-Powered Reminder and Habit-Tracking Apps:

AI-powered reminder and habit-tracking apps can assist individuals with OCD in managing their compulsive behaviors. These apps can provide reminders for medication, therapy sessions, and exposure exercises. Additionally, they can track progress and provide insights into habit patterns, helping individuals stay motivated and accountable.

Here are some working links and actual software and apps that you can explore for OCD management:

NOCD: You can find more information about the NOCD app and its features at their official website: NOCD

nOCD: You can learn more about the nOCD app and its functionalities on their website: nOCD

Woebot: You can download the Woebot app from the App Store or Google Play Store. Here is the link to their website for more information: Woebot

MindShift: You can download the MindShift app from the App Store or Google Play Store. For more details, you can visit their website: MindShift

Youper: You can download the Youper app from the App Store or Google Play Store. To learn more about its features, visit their website: Youper

Please note that availability may vary depending on your location and device. It's advisable to visit the respective app stores or the official websites for the most up-to-date information and to download the apps.

Chapter 50: The Future of AI in Anxiety Relief: Innovations and Possibilities

Introduction:

The future of anxiety relief holds exciting possibilities with the continued advancements in artificial intelligence (AI) technology. In this chapter, we will explore some potential innovations and possibilities for AI in anxiety relief.

Emotion Recognition AI:

AI algorithms can continue to improve in their ability to accurately recognize and interpret human emotions. This could lead to the development of AI-powered tools that can detect and respond to an individual's emotional state in real-time, offering personalized support and interventions.

Personalized AI Therapy:

AI has the potential to provide personalized therapy experiences tailored to an individual's specific needs and preferences. By analyzing data and feedback, AI algorithms can adapt therapy techniques, interventions, and content to optimize treatment outcomes.

Wearable AI for Real-time Support:

Advancements in wearable technology combined with AI can provide real-time support for anxiety management. Wearable devices equipped with AI algorithms can detect physiological markers of anxiety and provide immediate interventions, such as guided breathing exercises or calming prompts.

AI-Driven Virtual Support Communities:

AI can facilitate the creation of virtual support communities that connect individuals with similar anxiety experiences. AI algorithms can match individuals based on their needs, preferences, and goals, fostering a sense of belonging and providing a supportive network.

AI-Powered Early Intervention and Prevention:

AI algorithms can analyze various data sources, such as social media activity, sleep patterns, and physiological markers, to identify early signs of anxiety. This can enable early intervention and prevention strategies, helping individuals address anxiety before it becomes more severe.

Please note that the future possibilities mentioned in Chapter 50 are speculative and represent potential directions for AI in anxiety relief. As technology continues to evolve, new innovations and possibilities may emerge.

Here are some general examples and areas where AI is being explored for anxiety relief:

Emotion Recognition AI: Companies like Affectiva and Beyond Verbal are working on emotion recognition AI technology that can analyze facial expressions, vocal patterns, and other physiological signals to understand and respond to human emotions.

Personalized AI Therapy: Platforms like Woebot and Wysa are AI-powered chatbot apps that offer personalized therapy experiences by adapting their responses and interventions based on user input and feedback.

Wearable AI for Real-time Support: While specific AI-powered wearable devices for anxiety management may not be widely available, there are wearable technologies like smartwatches and fitness trackers that can monitor heart rate, sleep patterns, and stress levels, which can be used in conjunction with anxiety management techniques.

AI-Driven Virtual Support Communities: Online platforms and social networks like 7 Cups and Supportiv provide AI-driven matchmaking algorithms to connect individuals with similar experiences and provide a virtual support network.

AI-Powered Early Intervention and Prevention: Researchers are exploring the use of AI algorithms to analyze various data sources, including social media activity, to identify early signs of anxiety and provide targeted interventions. However, specific software or apps for this purpose may not be widely available yet.

Please keep in mind that these examples represent current trends and areas of exploration in AI for anxiety relief, and the specific tools and technologies may evolve over time. It's always recommended to stay updated with the latest research and developments in the field for the most accurate and up-to-date information.

Closing Address:

We hope that this book has provided you with valuable insights and information on the intersection of anxiety relief and artificial intelligence (AI). Throughout the chapters, we have explored various aspects of anxiety management and how AI can play a role in providing support, tools, and techniques to alleviate anxiety symptoms.

From understanding the causes and impact of anxiety to evaluating the benefits and limitations of AI-based solutions, we have delved into the potential of AI in enhancing traditional approaches to anxiety relief. We have discussed the importance of personalization, ethical considerations, privacy, and security when integrating AI into anxiety support systems.

By examining specific applications of AI, such as AI chatbots, virtual reality, biofeedback, and sleep solutions, we have showcased the diverse range of possibilities for using AI to manage anxiety. We have also explored how AI can be integrated with other approaches, such as professional therapy, human connection, self-care practices, and holistic approaches to provide comprehensive anxiety relief.

As we look towards the future, we have discussed potential innovations and possibilities for AI in anxiety relief. From emotion recognition AI to wearable technology, virtual support communities to early intervention and prevention strategies, the future holds exciting prospects for leveraging AI to better understand, manage, and prevent anxiety.

We encourage you to stay informed about the latest advancements in AI technology and its applications in anxiety relief. The field is rapidly evolving, and new tools, software, and apps may emerge that can further enhance anxiety management.

Remember, while AI can provide valuable support, it is important to seek professional help and consult with healthcare providers for a comprehensive treatment plan. Each individual's experience with anxiety is unique, and a personalized approach that combines human expertise with AI tools can lead to the most effective outcomes.

Thank you for joining us on this exploration of AI in anxiety relief. We wish you success in your journey towards managing anxiety and finding the support and tools that work best for you.

Warm regards,

Fellow Sufferer and Thriver